THE
MAGNESIUM
STEARATE

—— HANDBOOK ——

THE
MAGNESIUM
STEARATE

—————————— HANDBOOK ——————————

A Recommended Companion Guide for
Powder Technologists and Formulators

❖ *Complete Work on Polymorphism in Magnesium Stearate*

❖ *Effects on Powder Mixtures, Hardness, Dissolution*
   and Biopharmaceutic Classification System

PATRICK C.
OKOYE

℃iUniverse®

THE MAGNESIUM STEARATE HANDBOOK

iUniverse books may be ordered through booksellers or by contacting:

iUniverse
1663 Liberty Drive
Bloomington, IN 47403
www.iuniverse.com
1-800-Authors (1-800-288-4677)

ISBN: 978-1-5320-1111-5 (sc)
ISBN: 978-1-5320-1113-9 (hc)
ISBN: 978-1-5320-1112-2 (e)

Library of Congress Control Number: 2016918686

Print information available on the last page.

iUniverse rev. date: 12/15/2016

Preface

Magnesium stearate (MgSt) is widely used in cosmetic, food, and pharmaceutical formulations as lubricant in capsule and tablet manufacture at concentrations between 0.25% and 5%. A recent review of the top 200 prescription drugs showed over 50% contained magnesium stearate. This book covered a broad spectrum of concentration from 1% to 10% for the purpose of presenting their unique properties during powder rheology, tableting, and effect on drug dissolution. MgSt also has both scientific and economic significance given its wide application in global pharmaceutical manufacturing. An understanding of polymorphism (or pseudo polymorphism) in magnesium stearate including its impact on tablet lubrication process and drug dissolution, could provide valuable tool during excipient selection process for product development. Pre-formulation scientists spend a great deal of time reviewing excipients for new product development both *in silico* and on the bench. As a result, accurate selection of excipients, such as lubricants, could avoid potential issues with clinical batches, product scale-up, and product transfer during commercialization.

Patrick C. Okoye

Visit www.magnesium-stearate.com

Foreword

As magnesium stearate (MgSt) continues to be the excipient of choice for pharmaceutical solid oral dose blends its proper use can sometimes be diverted due to attractive claims associated with rectifying tablet quality issues. The best use of MgSt is commonly misunderstood and often misused particularly when tablet issues arise such as tool binding during the compression cycle. It is often utilized to address picking problems. Picking is the adherence of powder in the corners and/or island of a logo embossed on the punch face. Characters such as A, D and O and numerals such as 4, 6 and 8 are often problematic. If minor picking problems are not addressed properly then typical picking may escalate to a more serious tablet defect known as sticking. Sticking may result in unacceptable tablet appearance and in severe cases may cause weight and content uniformity issues. Hence, the utilization of MgSt as a quick and easy solution to simple tablet manufacturing problems may result in or contribute to not readily foreseeable problems with effectiveness of a given medicine.

Development and delivery of a pharmaceutical oral dosage blend demands a quality by design (QbD) approach. Understanding the assembly of the active pharmaceutical ingredient with its associated fillers, binders, lubricants, glidants and disintegrant requires a thorough knowledge of the function of each component and the impact of each component on the safety, integrity, strength, purity and quality of the tablet delivered to the patient. MgSt is one of the most popular lubricants utilized in the pharmaceutical tablet manufacturing industry. The physical properties of MgSt determine its impact on the properties of the bulk powder of which it is a component, the compression strength of tablets made with that powder and ultimately the stability and bioavailability of the therapeutic molecule being delivered to the patient. The reality is that MgSt has a variety of available polymorphs to go along with an array of particle size distributions. The lot to lot variability of these physical properties and others discussed in this book can impact the product being manufactured. A properly designed experimental assessment of different blend manufacturing techniques requires acknowledgement of these differences and the understanding of potential implications of this excipient variability.

This book offers the reader insight into the physical and chemical properties of a tablet component all too often overlooked in the design of the formulation. Dr. Patrick C. Okoye has invested a significant portion of his career as a pharmacist and researcher in pursuit of a comprehensive understanding of the role of MgSt in pharmaceutical dosage forms. Dr Patrick C. Okoye's work provides measurements of the chemical and physical properties of the different forms of MgSt along with an overview of the impact of MgSt on powder rheology. In addition, studies of the impact of MgSt on tablet physical properties and active pharmaceutical ingredient dissolution are provided. There is a wealth of information in this book and its references that will assist any formulator concerned with the selection and use of MgSt as a lubricant in a pharmaceutical, cosmetic or food presentation.

Dale Natoli DSc h.c.
President/Ceo Natoli Engineering

Dedication

*To all the pharmaceutical scientists who work
tirelessly to move the science forward*

Table of Contents

Chapter V

List of Figures

List of Tables

List of Appendices

Chapter I

In this chapter, the reader is presented
with the background on magnesium stearate
including some historical findings and challenges.
The reader is also introduced to the rheological,
biopharmaceutic and economic implications of
powder mixture lubrication

1.0 Overview

The influence of magnesium stearate ($C_{36}H_{70}MgO_4$, MW= 591.34) on blends and finished solid dosage products has presented significant challenges to drug manufacturing, including poor production efficiency and variability in drug disintegration and dissolution. Often, using inappropriate types and amounts of lubricants such as stearic acid, glyceryl behenate, sodium stearyl fumarate, boron nitride, and MgSt as release agents during blending or powder mixing, tends to compromise the physical attributes and quality of compressed tablets. Such deleterious effects are observed as disturbances in particle–particle interaction and tend to lead to variable powder flow, undesirable friability, high compression and ejection forces during tableting, and altered dissolution profiles [1-5]. As such, the amount, type, and duration of application of lubricants are often deemed as important factors to consider relative to the process acceptance and quality of finished goods. MgSt is widely used as a lubricant in the pharmaceutical industry. The advantages of MgSt over other lubricants include its high melting temperature, high lubricity at a low concentration, large covering potential, general acceptance as safe, non-toxicity, and its excellent stability profile. It is commercially available mainly in the mixed or undifferentiated form. Recently several polymorphic forms (MgSt anhydrate, MgSt-A; MgSt monohydrate, MgSt-M; and MgSt dihydrate, MgSt-D) have become available mainly for investigational purposes [6-8]. While the literature is replete with studies on powder lubrication with undifferentiated MgSt, it is, however, very scanty on the application and benefits of the individual polymorphic forms. As a result, little scientific information is available regarding the physical, molecular, and thermal characterization of these polymorphs.

MgSt is also used in the undifferentiated form as mixtures of the crystalline and amorphous forms of the hydrates in unknown ratios [9] Although lubricants may not qualify explicitly as flow agents, their application in aerosolization process, encapsulation, personal care products, and even as anti-caking and mold release agent in color cosmetics, has provided numerous benefits and increased popularity [10-11]. It had been suggested that the lubrication properties of pure MgSt depended on its moisture content and crystal structure [12]. For instance, it was reported that the water of hydration in the dihydrate form was more tightly bound than that in the trihydrate form [13]. It had also been shown that the transition from one polymorphic form to another was influenced by changes in temperature and humidity, and that the initial water content could be good parameter to describe the lubricating properties of the polymorphs, as opposed to the specific surface area. Similarly, it was also suggested that structural modification to the hydrate states of some MgSt polymorphs was a reversible process occurring only at high temperature and in the presence of moisture [14-17].

Although, these works showed much characterization of MgSt in blending or tableting processes, the authors alluded to the difficulty in isolating the individual polymorphs for any large-scale investigational work. They attributed the difficulty to the disproportionate reliance on powder diffraction in deciphering the various MgSt polymorphs. Other researchers, however, suggested that depending on the crystallization process, MgSt anhydrate, $C_{36}H_{70}MgO_4$, has been shown to convert reversibly to the trihydrate polymorphic form, even at room temperature and relative humidities $\geq 50\%$. They also maintained that depending on the temperature and percent relative humidity of the powder samples, the resultant MgSt product could be a combination of hydrates, anhydrate, and amorphous forms [18-20]. Also, other studies suggested that monohydrate and dihydrate forms of MgSt polymorphs are essentially stable at ambient storage conditions; and they do not convert to each other [7-8]. Hence, the current body of scientific literature seemed to suggest that the differences in performance of various commercially available MgSt might be uniquely tied to the degree of hydration and crystallization relative to advances in commercial crystallization processes.

1.1 Rheology of Powders

Many product and process development investigators still grapple with the selection of effective lubricant for their solid-dosage systems. Indeed, it is quite striking that the global industrial advances of the past half a century in areas of pharmaceutical manufacture still left behind many people from understanding the behavior of the most commonly used single ingredient in solid dosage formulations. Although many studies have been conducted to elucidate undifferentiated form of MgSt using X-ray Powder diffraction (XRD), limited application of other methods such as scanning electron microscopy (SEM), differential scanning calorimeter (DSC), melting point, moisture sorption isotherm (DVS), thermogravimetry (TGA), and compaction analysis have also been employed [21-24]. X-ray Powder diffraction (XRD) provides important powder crystalline patterns, additional information relating to lubricity profile, plasticization, densification, powder flow stability, permeability, covering potential, compaction, and any impact on dissolution is needed to elucidate the behavior of the polymorphs.

1.2 Dissolution and Biopharmaceutic Classification

Tablet dissolution failures are often attributed to poor performance of the drug substance *in vitro*, and could lead to rejection of formulation design; addition of excessive amount of surfactants to mimic solubilization *in vivo*; and possibly failure to justify biowaiver extension application under the Biopharmaceutics Classification System (BCS) [25-26]. Sadly, product and processing issues relating to tablet lubrication have persisted even when numerous investigators have attempted to understand the behavior of this single excipient, when it is used as lubricant [27].

The retarding effect of lubricants on the dissolution of model BCS Class I drug, salicylic acid, had been studied and was attributed to the hydrophobicity and concentration of the lubricants [28]. On the other hand, several independent investigators, including the U.S. Food and Drug Administration (FDA), have recognized the effects of excipients on the rate and extent of oral drug absorption especially for drug substances in BCS II and III [29]. Numerous studies have also attempted to identify the physical or chemical property of magnesium stearate that controls its lubricating role in tableting process. However, it has been suggested that such property might come from its covering potential or surface area [13-19]. Other studies attributed the effect to its hydrophobic nature or the presence of water of hydration in the mixed or undifferentiated forms of MgSt [20-23].

The main driver for such renewed interest in MgSt has been the global economic goal of reducing product rejection; conserve research and development funds from non-viable drug projects; and also, to mitigate the decline in manufacturing productivity [27]. As such, developing good understanding of the behavior of magnesium stearate is necessary to defining the properties of its polymorphic forms. Additionally, if any significant differences are observed between the commercially available polymorphs, elucidation of the underlining factors, even at physical, chemical, or molecular level, could be used to develop predictive models or solutions to the lubrication problems.

This book focused on solid-state characterization, powder rheology, atomic intensity of magnesium, and dissolution-effecting properties attributed to magnesium stearate polymorphs (anhydrate, monohydrate, and dihydrate) in powders and tablets. Thermal and spectroscopic analysis of the polymorphs were also evaluated. Powder behavior was evaluated using rheometric indicators such as permeability and basic flowability index, including density, porosity analysis, and lubricity index measurements. Finally, tablet characteristics such as compressional forces, as well as, atomic analysis using laser-induced spectroscopy were also evaluated.

Furthermore, this book focused on the behavior of three polymorphs of MgSt from surface physical chemistry and dissolution perspectives. The review employed dynamic vapor sorption, equilibrium binding, and particle–moisture interfacial tension in order to evaluate the effects of MgSt polymorphs on drug dissolution for immediate release dosage of APAP, that has high solubility and low permeability (BCS III) and NAPR, with low solubility and high permeability (BCS II) as model drugs.

A review of the top 200 prescription drugs showed that MgSt constituted approximately 54%, with lactose (as diluent) as a distant second at 38% as shown in Figure 1.

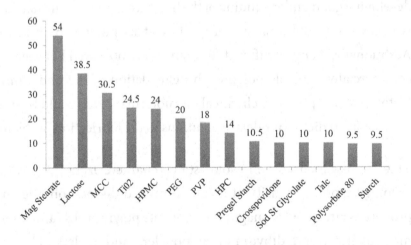

Figure 1: Percent Most Commonly Used Excipients in Top 200 Drugs (Ref: Mallinckrodt, Inc.)

Chapter II

In this chapter, the reader is presented
with ingredient (excipient-level) characterization
of the magnesium stearate polymorphs,
including solid-state, micromeritics,
thermal and electromagnetic wave analysis.

2.0 Excipient Characterization

MgSt polymorphs were characterized using several solid-state techniques including thermal conductivity, infra red spectroscopy, powder x-ray diffraction, thermogravimetry, differential scanning techniques, and dynamic vapor sorption.

2.1 Thermal Conductivity (TCi)

The property of materials to conduct heat is known as its thermal conductivity, k. This experimentation evaluated the ability of the MgSt polymorphs to conduct heat. Five samples of each MgSt polymorph were prepared and analyzed using thermal conductivity probe, TCi (C-Therm Technologies, Nova Scotia, Canada). Thermal conductivity of solid, pastes, and liquids can be measured rapidly in seconds using the TCi probe. The measurement temperature range was – 50 to 200 °C materials and the thermal conductivity values range from 0 to 100 W/mK. Sample amount in the range of 250 – 500 mg were placed in the test cell on the sensor and a standard weight were placed onto the sample so that it seats on the rim of the test cell.

Thermal Conductivity measurements were taken for the MgSt polymorphs and are shown in Table 1. Multiple measurements were taken for each polymorph and relative standard deviation values were obtained.

Test	MgSt polymorphs		
	Anhydrate	Monohydrate	Dihydrate
Thermal Conductivity, W/mK	0.053	0.048	0.050

Table 1: Thermal Conductivity Values for MgSt Polymorphs (Ref: PC Okoye, doctorate thesis)

The results from thermal conductivity analysis showed that MgSt-A has an average conductivity value of 0.053 W/mK (RSD 0.49%); the MgSt-M has average conductivity of 0.048 W/mK (RSD 0.47%); and MgSt-D has average conductivity of 0.050 W/mK (RSD 0.32%). The results showed that the three polymorphs have comparable thermal conductivities and the slight differences were not found to be significant enough to explain the differing behaviors of the polymorphs.

2.2 Infra Red Spectroscopy (FT-IR)

The object of infra red spectroscopy allows the measure of light absorption by materials at specific wavelength. The application of Fourier transform to infra red spectroscopy offers the advantage to measure multiple wavelengths and beams of light simultaneously in addition to high signal-to-noise ratio.

The FTIR Spectrometer (Spectrum 2, Perkin Elmer, Massachusetts, USA) was operated in single-beam mode using optical system with data acquisition over a total range of 4000 to 370 cm^{-1} with a best resolution of 0.5 cm^{-1} and lithium tantalate ($LiTaO_3$) as the mid infrared detector. Each sample was equilibrated at 25 °C under vacuum. The instrument was calibrated using known reference standard followed by background scanning to eliminate any interferences. Samples were mounted on the graphite prism and spectral data were collected and evaluated.

Using the raw material identification technique of FT-IR, additional experimentation was performed to evaluate any possible conversion of one polymorph to another within MgSt. Neat MgSt polymorphs (MgSt-A, MgSt-M and MgSt-D were exposed to 100% humidity condition at room temperature and FT-IR scans were collected. The samples were then re-dried and re-evaluated using FT-IR.

The results for MgSt-D from Figure 2A showed absorbance of differentiating functional groups at 3100 - 3300 cm^{-1} (O-H group) and in the 1500- 1700 cm^{-1} region (C-O group). The results indicated unique O-H stretching vibration at 3200 cm^{-1}, which is indicative of the presence of water molecules. The MgSt-D is the dihydrate form of MgSt and is believed to contain two molecules of water of hydration.

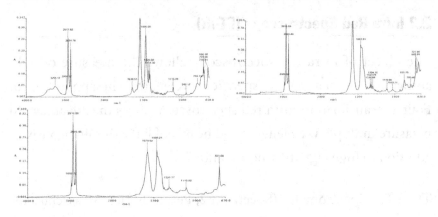

Clockwise: Figure 2A: Spectra Scan from FT-IR analysis of MgSt-D Polymorph. The scan gave prominent qualitative indication of available water of hydration; the presence of carbonyl groups in the 1600 cm^{-1} region.; and absence of bending vibration in the 850 cm^{-1} region. Figure 2B: Spectra Scan from FT-IR analysis of MgSt-M Polymorph. The scan showed reduced absorbance at 3200 cm^{-2} indicating presence of water, and presence of bending vibration in the 850 – 900 cm^{-1} region. Figure 3C Spectra Scan from FT-IR analysis of MgSt-A Polymorph. The scan gave showed absence water of hydration and absence of bending vibration in the 850 – 900 cm^{-1} region, an indication of differences in functional groups (Ref: PC Okoye, doctorate thesis).

Figure 2B shows the infra red spectra for MgSt-M. The results from the scan showed a small absorbance at 3200 cm^{-1} an indication of presence of water molecule. An additional vibration was observed at 875 cm^{-1}. The bending vibration in the 850 - 900 cm^{-1} region is indicative of presence of cis RCH=CHR alkene group [47]. The results from infra red analysis of MgSt-A in Figure 1C showed the absence of stretching vibration at 3200 cm^{-1} and also absence of bending vibration in the 850 – 900 cm^{-1} region. The results showed absence of water of hydration indicating that the material could be anhydrous in nature. These results showed some differing spectral characteristics between the MgSt polymorphs and could contribute to their unique behavior in pharmaceutical processing. Results from the inter-convertibility evaluation of MgSt polymorphs are presented in Figure 3 and shows distinct transitions.

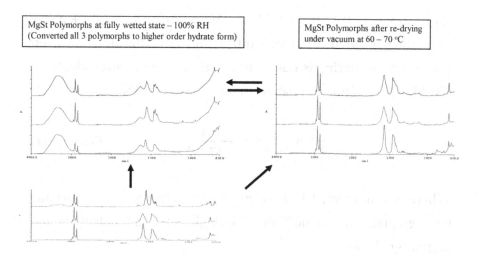

Figure 3: Annotated FT-IR scans of MgSt Polymorphs (Ref: PC Okoye, doctorate thesis).

The results in Figure 3 showed that the three polymorphs converted to higher order hydrate forms when fully exposed to 100% humidity condition at room temperature. The results also showed that upon re-drying under vacuum at 60 – 70 °C, the polyhydrate form (produced from MgSt-A and MgSt-D) and the "as is" MgSt-D polymorph converted to the anhydrous form (MgSt-A). However, polyhydrate form (produced from MgSt-M) reverted to the "as is" monohydrate form. These findings indicate that storage conditions such as temperature and humidity could be important for the performance of Magnesium stearate polymorphs in pharmaceutical processing environment.

2.3 Powder X-Ray Diffraction (pXRD)

The techniques of powder X-Ray diffraction enable the measure of scattered electromagnetic waves based on interaction with unpaired electrons. The pXRD patterns of MgSt polymorph samples were measured with a Rigaku closed beam X-ray diffractometer (Rigaku, Texas, USA) over the range of $2\theta = 2°$ to $40°$ and a $2°$/min scan speed, 2/3° slits, 0.3 mm at 45kV/200Ma as shown in Figure 4. X-ray diffraction is based on Bragg's diffraction or scattering of neutron waves. The scattering is due to interaction with unpaired electrons resulting to a diffraction pattern based on the relation:

$$d_{spacing} = \frac{n\lambda}{2\,Sin\,\theta}$$ Equation (1)

Where, n = interger; λ is wavelength of incident wave; d = spacing between planes in atomic lattice; θ is angle between incident ray and scattering planes.

Results from the diffraction patterns for the MgSt polymorphs showed that all 3 polymorphs exhibited unique atomic diffraction peaks within the neighborhood of 20 – 25° at 2θ as presented in Figure 4 (A, B, C).

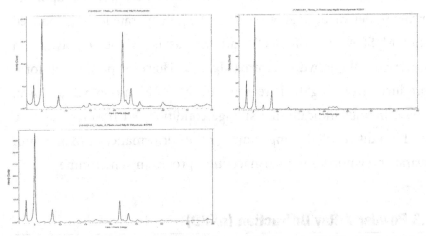

Clockwise Figure 4A: pXRD Diffraction pattern for MgSt-A Polymorph. The sharp peak within 22° at 2θ is characteristic of

MgSt-A and is related to its anhydrous nature. Figure 4B: pXRD Diffraction pattern for MgSt-M Polymorph. The absence of

any significant peak within 20 – 25° at 2θ is characteristic of MgSt-M and is believed to be related to is crystal structure.

Figure 4C: pXRD Diffraction pattern for MgSt-D Polymorph. The two reduced peaks within 20 - 25° at 2θ is characteristic

of MgSt-D and is believed to be related to its crystal structure nature (Ref: PC Okoye, doctorate thesis).

Figure 4A presents the diffraction pattern for MgSt-A showing significant intensity at 20 – 25° at 2θ. The peak intensity is an indication of the electron density. The diffraction pattern as presented in Figure 4B represents MgSt-M showing relative absence of any significant intensity within the neighborhood of 20 – 25° at 2θ. The absence of diffraction peaks in this area appeared to be unique to the monohydrate polymorph and is believe to contribute to its processing characteristics. Figure 4C represents the diffraction pattern for MgSt-D with characteristic peak within the neighborhood of 20 – 25° at 2θ. The results showed much lower intensity of the peak compared to MgSt-A, which is an indication of electron density. Additionally, the peak positions is a reflection of the translational symmetry, showing that MgSt-D and MgSt-A share the same structure except for the present of water of hydration in the dihydrate.

2.4 Thermogravimetric Analysis (TGA)

Thermogravimetric Analysis (TGA) is an evaluation of materials to determine the amount and rate of change in the weight of a material as a function of temperature. It is a technique used to characterize materials that exhibit weight loss or gain due to decomposition, oxidation, or dehydration. Based on the weight loss upon heating, the stoichiometry of hydrate and solvate compounds may be determined.

Samples of the MgSt polymorphs were analyzed using TA Instruments Q500 TGA (TA Instruments, Delaware). Each sample was loaded into an aluminum sample pan and heated from 25 °C to 250 °C using a heating rate of 10 °C / minute and nitrogen purge of 20 mL/min.

The results from the TGA traces are presented in Figure 5 (A, B, C) representing MgSt-A, MgSt-M and MgSt-D respectively. The traces indicate presence or absence of bound water of hydration in magnesium stearate.

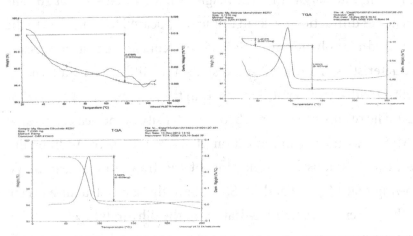

Clockwise Figure 5A: TGA trace for MgSt-A Polymorph. The trace showed absence of any significant water of hydration in the

anhydrate polymorph. Figure 5B: TGA trace for MgSt-M Polymorph. The trace showed presence of equivalent of one molecule of

water of hydration in the monohydrate polymorph. Figure 5C: TGA trace for MgSt-D Polymorph. The trace showed presence of

equivalent of two molecules of water of hydration in the dihydrate polymorph (Ref: PC Okoye, doctorate thesis).

Figure 5A shows the TGA trace for MgSt-A from 25 °C to 160 °C and indicated only a minimal water loss of 0.5766%. This represented possible unbound moisture in the excipient and also showed absence of water of hydration in the anhydrous polymorph. Stoichiometric analysis based on molecular weight of water (18g) and the molecular weight of MgSt (591.34 g) showed that 0.5766% loss represented only 3.41g loss well below the weight of water of hydration. Based on the stoichiometry, the 0.5766% loss is believed to unbound moisture in the material.

The TGA trace for MgSt-M is presented in Figure 5B and shows the exothermic transitions between 40 °C and and 110 °C. These transitions represented loss of unbound moisture up to 60 – 75 °C (mass of 0.4816%) and bound water of hydration up to 110 °C (mass of 2.880%) followed by indication of constant sample weight. A total of 3.3636% mass was lost representing a combination of unbound and bound moisture.

Stoichiometric analysis based on molecular weight of water (18g) and the molecular weight of MgSt (591.34 g) showed that 0.4816% loss represented only 2.93g loss well below the weight of water of hydration. Based on the stoichiometry, the 0.4816% loss is believed to unbound moisture in the material. Additionally, the loss of 2.880% at about 105 °C represented 17.55g loss. It is believed that based on experimental analysis, this amount appeared in close neighborhood to one molecule of water and is considered to be loss of one (bound) water molecule. Figure 5C shows the TGA trace for MgSt-D indicating the exothermic transition up to 125 °C. The transition is believed to represent loss of bound water of hydration (mass of 5.565%) followed by indication of constant sample weight.

Stoichiometric analysis based on molecular weight of water (18g) and the molecular weight of MgSt (591.34 g) showed that the loss of 5.565% at about 105 °C represented 34.91g loss. It is believed that based on experimental analysis, this amount appeared in close neighborhood to two molecules of water and are considered to be loss of two (bound) water molecules. The mass represented loss of two molecules of water from the dihydrate polymorph.

2.5 Differential Scanning Calorimeter (DSC)

2.5.1 Gibbs Energy and Enthalpy Determination

Differential scanning calorimetry is a technique that measures the difference in the amount of heat required to increase the temperature of a sample compared to a reference is measured. Differential scanning calorimetry was performed using TA Instruments Q200 DSC (TA Instruments, Delaware) Samples of weight 3-5 mg were tested in crimped aluminum pans, and an empty pan was used as a reference. The instrument was calibrated using pure indium sample. Sample testing was conducted from temperatures 25 ° to 150 °C at a heating rate of 2° C/min and nitrogen purge of 50 mL/min. Data acquisition and analysis were conducted using TA Instruments software.

Additional experimentation and analysis were performed using DSC to evaluate the possible existence of enantiotropism within the MgSt polymorphs. From thermal process, the change in Gibbs energy (ΔG) is given by:

$$\Delta G = \Delta H - T \Delta S \qquad \text{Equation (2)}$$

Also, the enthalpy change during such thermal process is given by:

$$\Delta H = \int_{T_1}^{T_2} C_p \, dT \qquad \text{Equation (3)}$$

At constant pressure, changes in entropy maybe calculated using:

$$\Delta S = \int_{T_1}^{T_2} \frac{C_p \, dT}{T} \qquad \text{Equation (4)}$$

Where ΔS is change in entropy (kJmol^{-1}); ΔH is change in enthalpy (kJmol^{-1}); C_p is heat capacity (JK^{-1}), and T is temperature in Kelvin. Knowing C_p and T from the DSC experimentation allows for the calculation of changes in entropy, enthalpy and Gibbs energy.

The results of the differential scanning calorimetry for the MgSt polymorphs are presented in Figure 6. These results show unique transitions for the three polymorphs providing significant evidence of differing characteristics. The DSC trace for the MgSt-A sample exhibited two primary transitions: first transition at 72 °C, appeared to be associated with loss of unbound moisture; the second transition at 119 °C, was associated with melting of samples. This water loss is consistent with the results from TGA which also showed slight moisture loss between 60 - 75 °C. The endothermic event at 119 °C clearly pointed to a melting process as indicated by the sharp peak followed by stable heat flow pattern.

The DSC trace for MgSt-M also exhibited two transitions: first indicated loss of bound moisture at 105 °C and the second indicated melting of sample at 125 °C. This water loss at 105 °C is consistent with the results from TGA which also significant moisture loss at about 105 °C. This water loss was marked by a relatively large enthalpy due to evaporation of released water. The endothermic event at 125 °C clearly pointed to a melting process as indicated by the sharp peak followed by stable heat flow pattern.

The DSC trace for MgSt-D, exhibits two transitions indicating loss of bound moisture at 89 °C and melting at 120 °C. This water loss at 89 °C is consistent with the results from TGA which also significant moisture loss at about 80 - 90 °C. The water loss was marked by a broad enthalpy due to evaporation of released water. The endothermic event at 120 °C clearly pointed to a melting process as indicated by the sharp peak followed by stable heat flow pattern. The results from the scans of MgSt-M and MgSt-D also suggested that the water in the monohydrate could be more tightly bound than in the dihydrate polymorph as shown by the higher melting point of 125 °C for the MgSt-M compared to MgSt-D melting point of 120 °C.

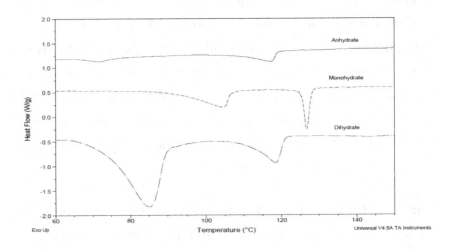

Figure 6: DSC Scans for MgSt Polymorphs. The scans showed melting point for anhydrous; the loss of water of hydration and melting point for the monohydrate; and the large transitional loss of water of hydration for the dehydrate (Ref: PC Okoye, doctorate thesis).

2.5.2 Evaluation of Monotropism and Enantiotropism

Results from the evaluation of possible monotropism or enantiotropism in MgSt polymorphs are presented in Figure 7. The results indicated that MgSt-D exhibited the highest change in Gibbs energy during the heating event as compared to the anhydrous and monohydrate polymorphs. This also appeared to indicate that the dihydrate form tends to be more spontaneous and might lose water of hydration quicker than the monohydrate.

The results also showed an overlap between the monohydrate (MgSt-M) and anhydrous form (MgSt-A) as detected at 335 K (62 °C). The results further indicated slight change in Gibbs energy for the MgSt-M from lower state to higher state prior to the melting points of 125 °C and 119 °C polymorphs. It is suspected that the monohydrate form exhibited more stability through this transition and appeared to be monotropic. This behavior appeared to be consistent with the results from the FT-IR analysis indicating that the MgSt-M could support a wider range of processing temperatures.

These results also suggest that with increasing temperature up to 350K, the MgSt-D possesses much lower ΔG (-23.35 kJmol^{-1}, Std Dev 0.06) than the MgSt-M (-18.85 kJmol^{-1}, Std Dev 0.04) and MgSt-A (-19.20 kJmol^{-1}, Std Dev 0.05). The possible explanation is that the dihydrate form is more spontaneous in behavior. Furthermore, changes in enthalpy suggest that at temperatures up to 350K, dihydrate form has slightly higher enthalpy (262 Jmol^{-1}, Std Dev 0.6) than either MgSt-A (225 Jmol^{-1}, Std Dev 0.6) and MgSt-M (208 Jmol^{-1}, Std Dev 0.6). Similarly, at the same temperature, MgSt-D has much higher heat capacity (15.08 J °C^{-1}, Std Dev 0.04) than MgSt-A (12.33 °C^{-1}, Std Dev 0.04), and MgSt-M (7.47 J °C^{-1}, Std Dev 0.004). This would suggest that MgSt-D presents higher energy barrier under thermal conditions than MgSt-A and MgSt-M.

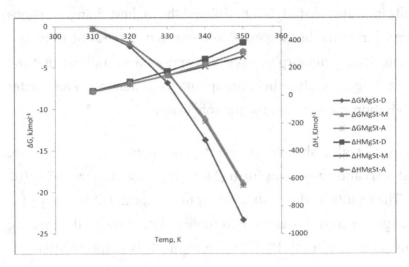

Figure 7: Plot for Evaluation of Monotropism and Enantiotropism in MgSt Polymorphs. The plot showed slight rise in

Gibb's energy at 335K (62 °C) from lower state to higher state for the monohydrate polymorph prior to its melting

point. Melting point, T_m: MgSt-A: 392K, MgSt-M: 398K, MgSt-D: 392K (Ref: PC Okoye, doctorate thesis).

2.6 Dynamic Vapor Sorption (DVS)

2.6.1 Water Activity (a_w) and Heat of Vaporization (ΔH)

The influence of water on the ability of MgSt polymorphs as boundary lubricants lends itself to the association between the amount of water (moisture content) that is held at a given energy state (water activity) at constant temperature and the adsorbing materials. This association is described by moisture sorption isotherms.

Samples were placed in high-density polyethylene sample cups and then placed in the test chamber. Each sample was initially vacuumed at 25 °C, 35 °C, and 45 °C for 7 days using a vacuum oven (Napco Precision Scientific, USA). The samples of MgSt polymorphs were then tested independently after equilibration at 25 °C using Aqua Lab Duo 4LTE (Decagon, Pullman, WA). From the Clausius-Clapeyron's relation for vapor pressure at different temperatures:

$$\ln\frac{P_1}{P_2} = \frac{\Delta H_{vap}}{R}(\frac{1}{T_2} - \frac{1}{T_1}) \qquad \text{Equation (5)}$$

Where P_1 and P_2 are the pressures (atm) at two temperatures T_1 and T_2 (in Kelvin); ΔH_{vap} is the enthalpic change of vaporization (J/mol); and R is the gas constant (Jmol^{-1}K^{-1}). (30)

Water activity, a_w, is defined as the ratio of partial pressure, p, of a substance to the saturated vapor pressure of pure water, p_0, at the same temperature as shown by:

$$a_w = \frac{p}{p_0} \qquad \text{Equation (6)}$$

Substituting a_w for P, in Equation (5), we obtain:

$$\ln\frac{a_{w1}}{a_{w2}} = \frac{\Delta H_{vap}}{R}(\frac{1}{T_2} - \frac{1}{T_1}) \qquad \text{Equation (7)}$$

Where ΔH_{vap}, is the heat of vaporization for the MgSt polymorph; a_{w1} and a_{w2} are water activity values of the material at temperatures, T_1 and T_2 respectively.

Results from the evaluation of water activity of the MgSt Polymorphs are presented in Table 2 and Figure 8. The mean water activity values indicated that for all three polymorphs the activity decreases with increase in temperature. Results from the analysis of water activity as a function of temperature provided the calculated heat of vaporization from Equations (6) and (7). Table 2 showed the linear relationship between water activity and temperature. The data shows that water activity of MgSt polymorphs decreases with increasing temperature. The data also showed that for all three polymorphs, the water activity decreases by half. It was observed that the water activity value for MgSt-A decreased from 0.35 at 25 °C to 0.17 at higher temperature of 45 °C. For MgSt-M, the water activity value decreased from 0.36 at 25 °C to 0.20 at higher temperature of 45 °C. Finally, the water activity value for MgSt-D decreased from 0.32 at 25 °C to 0.16 at higher temperature of 45 °C. Figure 6 depicts that relationship of water activity to temperature.

Temp (°C)	MgSt Polymorphs		
	MgSt A	MgSt M	MgSt D
25 C	0.3455 (±0.020)	0.3579 (±0.080)	0.3243 (±0.020)
35 C	0.2576 (±0.003)	0.2789 (±0.003)	0.2437 (±0.003)
45 C	0.1734 (±0.003)	0.2002 (±0.001)	0.1604 (±0.003)

Table 2: Evaluation of Water Activity (a_w) for MgSt Polymorphs (Ref: PC Okoye, doctorate thesis)

The enthalpy of vaporization for MgSt polymorphs from the non-isothermal events were obtained using Equation 7, as shown in Figure 8 for the individual polymorphs.

The enthalpy of vaporization was calculated for each polymorph by plotting the natural log of water activity of the temperature (in Kelvin). The polymorphs showed different enthalpies of vaporization as calculated from the slope of the plots. The MgSt-A showed ΔH –27.157 kJ/mol with $R^2 = 0.9927$. The MgSt-D gave ΔH –27.733 kJ/mol with $R^2 = 0.9990$. Finally, the MgSt-M gave ΔH –22.885 kJ/mol with $R^2 = 0.9934$.

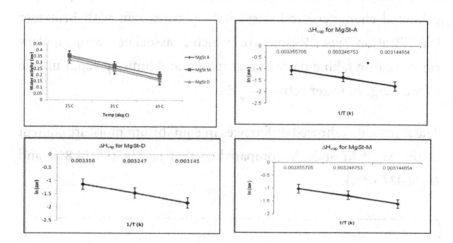

Clockwise Figure 8A: Plot for Water Activity and Temperature for MgSt Polymorphs. The plots showed the change in water activity for the polymorphs as a function of temp. Figure 8B: Plot for Natural Log of A_w and Temperature (K) for MgSt-A; product of the slope and gas constant (8.314 Jmol⁻¹K⁻¹) gives the ΔH_vaporization. Figure 8C: Plot for Natural Log of A_w and Temperature (K) for MgSt-M; product of the slope and gas constant (8.314 Jmol⁻¹K⁻¹) gives the ΔH_vaporization. Figure 8D: Plot for Natural Log of A_w and Temperature (K) for MgSt-D; product of the slope and gas constant (8.314 Jmol⁻¹K⁻¹) gives the ΔH_vaporization (Ref: PC Okoye, doctorate thesis).

2.6.2 Adsorption and Desorption Isotherms

Results from dynamic vapor adsorption are shown in Figure 9 indicating consistent moisture content at relatively low water activity (a_w) below 0.50 a_w for MgSt-A, MgSt-M, and MgSt-D. The isotherms showed sharp increase in moisture uptake for the polymorphs beyond 0.75 a_w. The results pointed to changes in effective relative humidity beyond equilibrium moisture conditions.

On the other hand, desorption curves for the polymorphs indicated greater tendency for moisture loss (evaporation) resulting in hysteresis between 0.55 a_w and 0.85 a_w, with MgSt-M showing slower but prolonged event. Figure 9 also depicted the several components of the wetting and drying patterns of MgSt polymorphs with the associated hysteresis. The results showed that the MgSt polymorphs exhibited characteristic hysteresis loop consistent with Brunauer Classification *Type IV* isotherm, which is associated with capillary condensation taking place in mesopores, and limiting vapor uptake over a range of water activity, a_w [52].

The results also showed differences in equilibrium moisture content of the MgSt-M at 3.2% compared to that of MgSt-A (4.8%) and MgSt-D (5.3%).

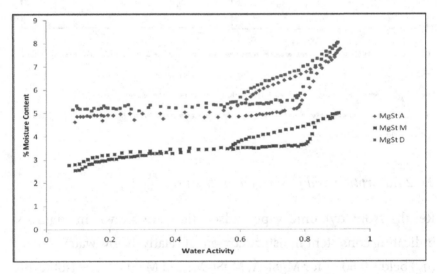

Figure 9: Plot for % Moisture Content and Water Activity for MgSt Polymorphs. The isotherms showed the

sorption (upward) and desorption (downward) curves for the polymorphs as developed from the moisture

content at various water activity values in anti-clockwise direction. The hysteresis is indicated by the pocket

between the upward and downward curves (Ref: PC Okoye, doctorate thesis).

2.6.3 Binding Constants and Monolayer values

The moisture sorption isotherm of products can be described by numerous mathematical models with two or more parameters. The monolayer model is described by Langmuir model while the multilayer adsorption is described by numerous models [30-32]. The adsorption of moisture unto multilayer surfaces is believed to follow the *Brunauer-Emmett-Teller* (BET) model. Similarly, we will make the assumption that adsorption of moisture unto MgSt particles follow the BET multilayer model.

The samples of MgSt polymorphs were tested independently at 25 °C using Aqualab Vapor Sorption Analyzer (Decagon, Pullman, WA). Each sample was initially vacuumed at 40 °C for 72 hours using a vacuum oven (Napco Precision Scientific, USA). Samples were then placed in a stainless steel cup, which was tared at the beginning of the test. The samples were subsequently dried down (desorption) to a water activity of 0.1, and then hydrated (adsorption) to a water activity of 0.9, and finally re-dried to a water activity of 0.1. Constant flow rate was maintained for the hydrated and desiccated air throughout the runs.

An equilibrium kinetic derivation of a multilayer model based on simple deposition of successive monolayers of an adsorbate (in this case, water molecules) on the adsorbent (MgSt) at constant temperature is presented. The assumptions in this model include presence of saturable open sites with reversible non-specific adsorption; there exist no interaction or reaction between the powder and moisture; and also, that the rate of free site occupation equals the rate of generation of open sites as described by:

$$a_0 P S_0 = b_0 S_1 e^{-E_B/RT} \qquad \text{Equation (8)}$$

Similarly, for S_1, S_2 and S_3, in equilibrium,

$$a_1 P S_1 = b_1 S_2 e^{-E_V/RT} \qquad \text{Equation (9)}$$

$$a_2 P S_2 = b_2 S_3 e^{-E_V/RT} \qquad \text{Equation (10)}$$

Where a_0, a_1, a_2, b_0, b_1, b_2, represent equivalent pre-exponential functions; R is the gas constant (8.314 J/mol K); and T is temperature (K); P is the partial pressure of the adsorbate; and S is the number of sites available on the adsorbent to be occupied; E_B, E_V, represent gas-solid and gas-gas binding energies respectively. Assume that for multilayer model: S_0 (unoccupied site) and S_1 (occupied site) are in equilibrium; S_1 and S_2 (occupied site) are in equilibrium; and also, S_2 and S_3 (occupied site) are in equilibrium. Hence, the values of S_1, S_2 and S_3 can be expressed as:

Assume,

$$X = \frac{a_1}{b_1} P e^{-E_B/RT} \qquad \text{Equation (11a)}$$

and

$$Y = \frac{a_0}{b_0} P e^{-E_B/RT} \qquad \text{Equation (11b)}$$

Then,

$$S_1 = \frac{a_0}{b_0} P e^{-E_B/RT} S_0 = Y S_0 \qquad \text{Equation (12)}$$

Similarly,

$$S_2 = \frac{a_1}{b_1} P e^{-E_V/RT} S_1 = X S_1 \qquad \text{Equation (13)}$$

and

$$S_3 = \frac{a_2}{b_2} P e^{-E_V/RT} S_2 = X S_2 \qquad \text{Equation (14)}$$

Dividing Equation (11b) by Equation (11a),

$$C = \frac{Y}{X} = \frac{a_0}{b_0} \cdot \frac{b_1}{a_1} e^{(E_B - E_V)/RT} = e^{\Delta E/RT} \qquad \text{Equation (15)}$$

Equation (15) represents the binding constant during adsorption and desorption. Substituting Y in terms of CX in Equations (12), (13), and (14), we obtain:

$$S_1 = Y S_0 = C X S_0 \qquad \text{Equation (16)}$$

$$S_2 = X S_1 = C X^2 S_0 \qquad \text{Equation (17)}$$

$$S_3 = X S_2 = C X^3 S_0 \qquad \text{Equation (18)}$$

Hence,

$$S_n = CX^n S_0 \qquad \text{Equation (19)}$$

For m molecules adsorbed, we can express the function as an infinite geometric progression:

$$m = \sum_{i=1}^{\infty} nS_n = \sum_{i=1}^{\infty} nCX^n S_0 = CS_0 \sum_{i=1}^{\infty} nX^n \qquad \text{Equation (20)}$$

Similarly, for a saturated monolayer, m_0, number of moles adsorbed can be represented by:

$$m_0 = S_0 + S_1 + \ldots = S_0 + \sum_{i=1}^{\infty} S_n = S_0 + \sum_{i=1}^{\infty} CS_0 X^n = S_0 \left[1 + C \sum_{i=1}^{\infty} X^n \right] \text{Equation (21)}$$

Dividing Equation (20) by Equation (21) and solving algebraically, we obtain:

$$\frac{m}{m_0} = \frac{CX}{(1-X)[1+(C-1)X]} \qquad \text{Equation (22)}$$

Where X (also known as water activity) represents the ratio of partial pressure of the adsorbate to the partial pressure of the pure substance and can be represented by:

$$a_w = \frac{p}{p_0} = X \qquad \text{Equation (23)}$$

We can now re-arrange Equation (22) to obtain the multilayer model of BET as shown by:

$$m = \frac{a_w m_0 C}{(1-a_w)[1+a_w(C-1)]} \qquad \text{Equation (24)}$$

Where m is the moisture content in g/g solids; a_w, is water activity; m_0, is the moisture content of monolayer in g/g solids. BET model is typically applicable up to 0.5 a_w [30, 32].

Experimental application of the BET multilayer model involves obtaining some initial values of water activity, a_w, with corresponding moisture content values, m. The analytical method involves linearization of Equation 24 to obtain:

$$\frac{[1+a_w(c-1)]}{m_0 c} = \frac{a_w}{(1-a_w)m} \qquad \text{Equation (25)}$$

Finally,

$$\frac{a_w}{(1-a_w)m} = a_w \left[\frac{c-1}{m_0 c}\right] + \frac{1}{m_0 c} \qquad \text{Equation (26)}$$

Where a plot of $\frac{a_w}{(1-a_w)m}$ versus a_w gives a straight line with slope as $\left[\frac{c-1}{m_0 c}\right]$ and the intercept as $\frac{1}{m_0 c}$. The BET parameters, m_0 and C, were experimentally obtained as $m_0 = \frac{1}{slope + \text{int} ercept}$ and $C = \frac{1}{\text{int} ercept * m_0}$.

2.6.4 Binding Energy (ΔE) of MgSt polymorphs and Moisture

The binding or surface energy for lubricant-moisture behavior was estimated from the BET Plot Equation (26) using water activity values from $0.1a_w$ to $0.5a_w$, representing the monolayer phase of the adsorption isotherm. We can further re-arrange Equation (15) to obtain:

$$\ln C = \frac{\Delta E}{RT} \qquad \text{Equation (27)}$$

$$\Delta E = RT \ln C \qquad \text{Equation (28)}$$

The results of binding energy (ΔE) analysis under isothermal condition for MgSt polymorphs are shown in Table 3. The results also indicated that the surface interaction energies differed from one polymorph to another with MgSt-M having a large value in particle-particle binding energy of 13,857 J mol[-1], and MgSt-D and MgSt-A showing lower binding energy of 4,995 J mol[-1] and 2,568 J mol[-1] respectively.

These results showed that the surface chemistry of MgSt polymorphs is influenced by their association with moisture under isothermal conditions. The determination of BET parameters for MgSt polymorphs could help to elucidate the effect of the surface phenomenon of MgSt on the dissolution of immediate release dosage forms, especially BCS Class II and III [52]. The binding constant, C, was found to differ significantly between the MgSt-M (C = 268.6), MgSt-A (C = 7.51), and MgSt-D (C = 2.82). This difference was attributed to the unique sorption behavior of the monohydrate form as shown by the BET plot < 0.5 a_w. The initial steady incline at low water activity for MgSt-M seemed to suggest low level micropore influence during the monolayer-multilayer formation. This effect was, however, not observed on the MgSt-A and MgSt-D forms. The monolayer values, m_0, for the polymorphs were found to be significantly different between MgSt-M (2.7 g/g solids), MgSt-A (25.1 g/g solids) and MgSt-D (26.1 g/g solids), as shown in Table 3. This supports the finding that interfacial surface energy for lubricant-moisture association for MgSt-M (13.9 kJ/mol) was much higher than those of MgSt-A (5 kJ/mol) and MgSt-D (2.6 kJ/mol) [31]. The divergent behavior of the MgSt-M when compared to those of MgSt-A and MgSt-D appeared to be related to these surface chemical characteristics.

2.6.5 Interfacial Tension (γ) of MgSt polymorphs and Moisture

The molecular relationship between solid–liquid interface may be described by the changes in surface energy (ΔE) due to non-expansion work. The deposition of monolayer of moisture on the lubricant molecules creates an interfacial tension following the Young-Laplace expression [33]:

$$\Delta E = \gamma A \qquad \text{Equation (29)}$$

Where ΔE is the surface or binding energy of the monolayer; γ is the molecular interfacial tension; and A is the molecular cross sectional area. If we assume monolayer saturable sites with each molecule of water spreading across the powder particle, then spatial separation between two water molecules is given by:

$$\left(\frac{V}{N} \right)^{\frac{1}{3}} \qquad \text{Equation (30)}$$

where V is the molar volume (18.02×10^{-6} m^3); and N is Avogadro's number (6.02×10^{23}).

$$\left(\frac{18.02x10^{-6}m^3}{6.02x10^{23}}\right)^{\frac{1}{3}} = \left(30.00x10^{-30}m^3\right)^{\frac{1}{3}} \approx 3.10x10^{-10}m \quad \text{Equation (31)}$$

The cross-sectional area of water molecule is then derived as:

$$A_{H_2O} = 3.10x10^{-10}m * 3x10^{-10}m = 9.64x10^{-20}m^2 \approx 1.00x10^{-19}m^2$$

If we assume non-interactive particle–particle behavior as espoused by BET, then the molecular interfacial tension between MgSt powder and water molecules could be estimated from the binding or surface energy at the saturable sites as given by:

$$\gamma = \frac{\Delta E}{N_{Avogadro}} * \frac{1}{A_{H_2O}} \quad \text{Equation (32)}$$

Where ΔE is monolayer binding or surface energy; $N_{Avogadro}$ is the Avogadro's number, ($6.02x10^{23} \, molecules / mol$); A_{H_2O} is the cross-sectional area of water molecule ($1.06x10^{-19} \, m^2$).

The results of analysis of interfacial tension (γ) between lubricant and moisture are presented in Table 3. The MgSt-M was found to show higher interfacial tension value of 217.2 dyne cm^{-1} compared to MgSt-A (78.5 dyne cm^{-1}) and MgSt-D (40.4 dyne cm^{-1}). The significance of this finding is that the potential of over-lubrication could be higher when MgSt-M is employed as lubricant indicating high interfacial tension from the MgSt-M – moisture (217.2 dyne cm^{-1}) and drugs with low solubility.

2.6.6 Determination of BET Parameters (m_0 and C)

Figure 10 (Top, Middle, Bottom) show the estimated results of BET parameters based on analysis of the slopes and intercepts. The binding constant (C) values were obtained as 268.6 (MgSt-M), 7.51 (MgSt-A), and 2.82 (MgSt-D). The monolayer contents were calculated as 2.7 g/g solids (MgSt-M), 25.1 g/g solids (MgSt-A), and 26.1 g/g solids (MgSt-D).

The results indicated an inverse relationship between the binding constant and monolayer contents. The linearity, R^2, is a measure of the fitness of the plot to the monolayer model of the BET as shown in Table 3. These results also suggest that the monohydrate form tend to be less spontaneous than both the anhydrous and dihydrate forms. These results also support the findings from FT-IR analysis, TGA, and DSC analysis suggesting that water of hydration in the monohydrate might be more tightly bound than that in the dihydrate.

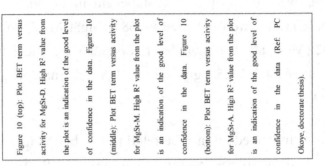

Figure 10 (top): Plot BET term versus activity for MgSt-D. High R^2 value from the plot is an indication of the good level of confidence in the data. Figure 10 (middle): Plot BET term versus activity for MgSt-M. High R^2 value from the plot is an indication of the good level of confidence in the data. Figure 10 (bottom): Plot BET term versus activity for MgSt-A. High R^2 value from the plot is an indication of the good level of confidence in the data (Ref: PC Okoye, doctorate thesis).

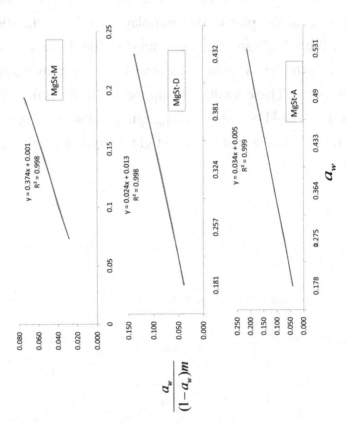

BET Parameters at 25 °C	MgSt polymorphs		
	Monohydrate	Anhydrous	Dihydrate
Initial moisture content at 25 °C	3.4000	5.3000	5.5000
Binding Constant, C	268.60	7.51	2.82
Monolayer, m_0 (g/g solids)	2.70	25.10	26.10
R^2 on BET parameters	0.9985	0.9994	0.9987
Binding Energy, ΔE (J/mol)	13,857	4,995	2,568
Estimated Interfacial Tension, γ (dyne cm^{-1})	217.20	78.50	40.40

Table 3: Thermodynamic and Moisture Sorption parameters (Ref: PC Okoye, doctorate thesis)

2.7 Other Miscellaneous Tests

Evaluation of the polymorphs was performed using particle size analysis, as well as, a review of current specifications of the undifferentiated form of MgSt.

2.7.1 Particle Size Analysis of MgSt Polymorphs

Particle size analysis of MgSt polymorphs was performed using Mastersizer 3000 laser diffraction system (Malvern Instruments Ltd, Malvern, Worcestershire, United Kingdom) equipped with a 63 mm lens (size range from 10.0 nm – 3.5 mm) and a stirred cell. The instrument uses a technique of laser diffraction to measure the size of dispersed particles by measuring the scattered laser beam intensity as the beam passes through a dispersed sample. Samples of MgSt polymorphs were prepared by dispersing each polymorph in mineral oil following by placement in the test chamber. The results show that MgSt-M has slightly lower particle size of 10.6 µm at d_{50}, followed by MgSt-D with 14.3 µm at d_{50}. The MgSt-A has the largest particle size of 15.1 um at d_{50}. These results show slight difference between the polymorphs. However, it is not clear whether this slight difference in particle size is significant to influence the behavior of the MgSt polymorphs when used as single or mixed ratio lubricants.

2.7.2 MgSt (undifferentiated form)

Typically, MgSt is available in the mixed form in unknown ratios, for pharmaceutical processing. Although MgSt polymorphs are commonly available, the mixed form remains the single widely used form and also easily found in reference and compendial documents.

Table 4 showed that typical specifications listed for MgSt by manufacturers and vendors.

Product Code	MgSt (mixed form)
Stearic: Palmitic	65:35
Particle Size, 50th %	10.5-16.5 microns
Particle Size, 90th %	35 micron max
Specific Surface Area	5-10 m²/g
Apparent Density	0.08-0.17 g/cc
Tapped Density	0.21-0.33 g/cc
Free Fatty Acid	2.0% max
Identification (FCC)	54⁰C min
Assay (MgO) (FCC)	6.8-8.3%
Appearance	Fine, white powder
ID (Magnesium)	Meets requirement

Table 4: Magnesium Stearate Specifications (Reference: Mallinckrodt, Inc.)

Chapter III

In this chapter, the reader is presented
with powder mixture (blend) level characterization
using prototype mixtures to evaluate rheological patterns,
lubricity indices, and micromeritics

3.0 Powder Mixtures Characterization

Powder Mixtures comprising several excipients, drug substance and varying concentrations of MgSt polymorphs were evaluated. The mixtures were characterized using techniques including bulk and tapped density techniques, powder compaction, lubricity index determination, powder permeability and flowability.

3.1 Prototype Formulation 1

Powder mixtures of direct compression formulations employed in the study contained acetaminophen, USP (5%); microcrystlline cellulose, NF (72%); lactose monohydrate, USP (22%); and MgSt (1%). Experimental design in Table 5 shows the various ratios of MgSt polymorphs used in the formulations. Each binary combination of MgSt polymorphs was pre-mixed by hand in a polybag for 2 minutes prior to use as lubricant in the blend.

3.1.1 Experimental Designs

The experimental designs for MgSt polymorphs are illustrated in Table 5.

Formula	MgSt-A[1] %	MgSt-M[2] %	MgSt-D[3] %	%Total MgSt[4]
D1	0.50	0.50		1.00
D2	0.25	0.75	---	1.00
D3	0.75	0.25		1.00
D4	0.50		0.50	1.00
D5	0.25	---	0.75	1.00
D6	0.75		0.25	1.00
D7		0.50	0.50	1.00
D8	---	0.25	0.75	1.00
D9		0.75	0.25	1.00
DA01	1.00	---		1.00
DM01		1.00	---	1.00
DD01	---	---	1.00	1.00
Un-lubricated	Control			

[1] % MgSt-A (anhydrate) in the blend formula; [2] % MgSt-M (monohydrate) in the blend formula; [3] % MgSt-D (dihydrate) in the blend formula; [4] Total % MgSt in the blend formula

Table 5: Experimental Designs -Ratios of Magnesium Stearate (MgSt) Polymorphs (Ref: PC Okoye, doctorate thesis)

3.2 Rheometry

Powder rheometry analysis was conducted using FT4 Rheometer (Freeman Technologies (Welland, UK) to evaluate permeability, percent compressibility, and flow energy of the mixtures. The instrument was calibrated using three standards protocol for force, torque and height calibration to monitor density values.

3.2.1 Permeability of Powder Mixtures

Permeability was measured as pressure drop across powder beds against a varying applied normal pressure (1-15 kPa) while the air velocity through the bed was maintained at constant rate of 2mm/s.

Each blend was tested eight (8) times under pressure. The setup used a 50 mm x 85 ml split vessel, 48 mm blade and a vented piston to compress the sample under increasing normal stresses whilst at the same time, air was passed up through the vessel at a constant flow rate. Permeability is a measure of how easily material can transmit a fluid (e.g. air) through its bulk. The air pressure drop across the powder bed (i.e. the resistance to air flow through the powder) is measured for each applied normal stress. The greater the pressure drop, the less permeable the powder becomes. Permeability (K) can be derived using Darcy's Law [34]:

$$K = \frac{Q\,\mu L}{A\left(P_a - P_b\right)} \qquad \text{Equation (33)}$$

Where, Q is air volume per unit time (cm^3/s), K is Permeability (cm^2), A is cross-sectional area of powder bed (cm^2), $P_a - P_b$ is pressure drop across powder bed (Pa), μ is air viscosity (Pa.s), L is Length of powder bed (cm).

Results from the permeability analysis are shown in Figure 11. The results showed that lubrication of powder blends with MgSt generally decreased the permeability values when compared to unlubricated blends. The results also showed that the unlubricated blends (unlubed) had the highest permeability followed by the blends lubricated with MgSt-A (DA01) and MgSt-D (DD01) suggesting the effect of intermolecular packing or arrangement. Data analysis using *paired t-test* showed the decrease in permeability for lubricated powder mixtures to be significant (p<0.005). The blend containing MgSt-M (DM01) alone, showed the lowest permeability. This suggested that blends containing MgSt-M required higher pressure (than those containing either MgSt-A or MgSt-D) in order to establish air-flow through powder bed as very small or limited number of channels is present between particles.

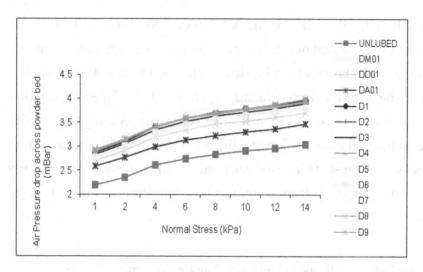

Figure 11: Permeability (air pressure drop) for non-lubricated and lubricated blend. The non-lubricated powder

blend showed the lowest drop in air pressure compared to the single polymorphs (Ref: PC Okoye, doctorate thesis).

3.2.2 Basic Flowability Energy (BFE) and Flow Stability Index (FSI)

Basic flowability energy (BFE) also known as powder flow energy (mJ), is the energy required to establish a flow pattern in a conditioned, precise volume of powder obtained through a downward anti-clockwise motion of the blade. This energy was evaluated at tip speed of 100 mm per second using a 50 mm x 160 ml vessel, 48 mm blade. Following the method as previously developed, seven (7) tests were performed on previously conditioned blends. The flow stability index (FSI) is a measure of powder flowability and is defined by the ratio of Test 7 to Test 1 [35]. Any change may be attributed to factors such as attrition, segregation or even electrostatic charge. Sample with a flow stability index of less than unity indicates poor flow and also, that the powder blend becomes freer flowing as a result of the testing, possibly due to rounding of the particles [36].

Results of the flow stability index (SI) results are shown in Table 7. The results showed that non-lubricated blends required the lowest energy to flow at 100 mm/s than lubricated blends. The results also showed that the non-lubricated blend experienced the largest reduction in flow energy (up to 89 mJ) after seven consecutive tests, hence resulting to the lowest flow stability index of 0.83. This indicated that the non-lubricated blend experienced significant reduction in energy due to the attrition from rounding and smoothing of the particles in motion (p<0.005).

3.2.3 Bulk and Tapped Density of Powder Mixtures (ρ_{Bulk}, ρ_{Tapped})

Each powder sample was accurately weighed to twenty grams (20 g) using a calibrated balance, (Sartorious Basic, Model B1-205). The powder was carefully poured into a tilted 100-mL graduated cylinder to avoid compaction. The cylinder was then dropped from a height of 1 inch onto a hard surface three times at 2 second intervals and subsequently the bulk volume of each powder blend was measured. Tapped volume of each powder was obtained by securing the cylinder onto a Vanderkamp Tap Density Tester (VanKel Industries, Edison, NJ) and the tapped volume was measured after 2000 taps. Bulk and Tapped densities was calculated from the ratios of mass and volume [37].

$$Density, \rho = \frac{mass}{volume}$$ Equation (34)

3.2.4 True Density (ρ_{True}) and Total Porosity (ε_{Total}) of Powder Mixtures

Powder samples were analyzed using Quantachrome – Ultrapycnometer 1000 (Quantachrome Instruments, Boynton, FL). Each sample was equilibrated under helium gas flow for at least 10 minutes. Five runs of each sample were conducted using medium pycnometer cell. The total porosity, ε_{Total}, is the sum of pores within particles and the relative void volume. It is also expressed as the ratio of the bulk density and the true density:

$$\varepsilon_{Total} = 1 - \frac{\rho_{bulk}}{\rho_{true}} \qquad \text{Equation (35)}$$

Where ρ_{bulk} is the bulk density; and ρ_{true} is the true density of the powder or material under inspection previously obtained using helium pycnometry [38].

Bulk and true density measurements were performed on the MgSt polymorphs and the results are presented in Table 6. Multiple measurements were taken for each polymorph. The bulk and true density results showed comparable values for all three polymorphs. The calculated porosity also presented comparable results an indication that the total pore sizes may not completely describe the characteristics of the polymorphs [50-51].

The results in Figure 12 showed that the total porosities for the blends indicate some differences in the packing of the particle under blended state. The results show that blends lubricated with MgSt-D or combinations of MgSt-D and MgSt-A tend to be more loosely packed than the blends containing MgSt-M. Although the differences are relatively small between the batches, they tend to suggest that the total porosity could be influenced by type of polymorphs or the MgSt mixed ratio used.

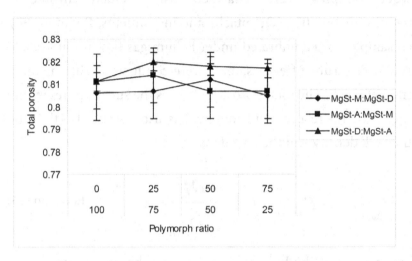

Figure 12: Total Porosity of batches lubricated with MgSt polymorphs (n=3; RSD <3.4%); MgSt-M:MgSt-D ratio means 100%:0% from left to right on x-axis; MgSt-A: MgSt-M ratio means 100%:0% from left to right on x-axis; and MgSt-D: MgSt-A ratio means 100%:0% from left to right on x-axis (Ref: PC Okoye, doctorate thesis).

Test	MgSt Polymorph		
	Anhydrate	Monohydrate	Dihydrate
Bulk Density g/mL	0.120 (±0.008)	0.110 (±0.008)	0.130 (±0.008)
True Density g/Ml	1.026 (±0.002)	1.052 (±0.002)	1.042 (±0.003)
Calculated Total Porosity	0.883 (±0.008)	0.895 (±0.008)	0.875 (±0.008)

Table 6: Density and Porosity Analysis of MgSt polymorph (Ref: PC Okoye, doctorate thesis)

3.2.5 Compaction of Powder Mixtures containing MgSt Polymorphs

Compacts were produced on a single punch press (MTCM-1, Globe Phama, NJ USA), using standard B-tooling flat punch with diameter 0.375 inch. Each compact weighed approximately 1000 mg. A pressure of 4,000 psi, was applied using a manual lever and held for 60 seconds. The compaction pressure was selected when no further reduction in thickness was observed when the un-lubricated blend was subjected to increasing pressure up to 4,000 psi. Each blend was accurately weighed and compacted. The compacts were subsequently ejected and thickness measured using a graduated thickness measure (B. C. Ames, Mass, USA). Assuming a cylindrical dimension, the volume of each compact was calculated as a product of the area of the compact face (punch face area or radial) and the thickness of the compact (axial) [39-40].

3.2.6 Lubricity Index, Ω

Lubricity index, Ω, has been proposed as a measure of the tendency of a material or powder mixture to over-lubricate [1, 8] Lubricity of powders is influenced more by the properties of lubricants employed than those of other ingredients [45]. The strength of a compact is directly related to the applied pressure. As compacts are formed and broken, fragmentation of the particles tend to create new bonding sites and create radial and axial strength relative to the newly formed compact. The lubricity index was proposed from the exerted radial pressure as depicted below [1, 8]:

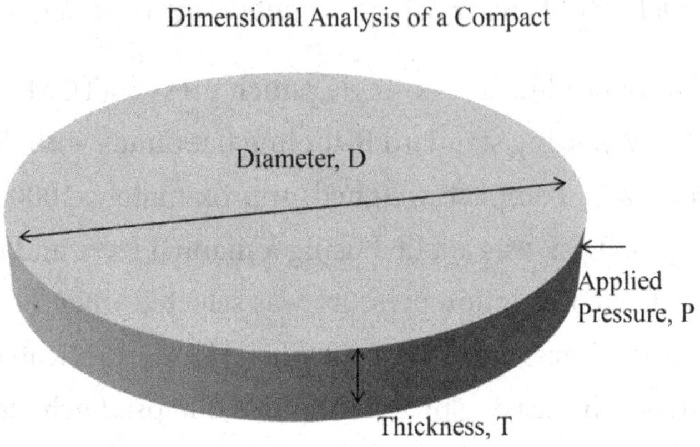

Dimensional Analysis of a Compact

Figure 13: Annotated Cylindrical disc

Consider a compact as a cylindrical structure whose surface area, A, is given by:

$$A = \pi DT + 2\pi r^2$$ Equation (36)

and the applied radial pressure, P, is given by:

$$P = \frac{Force}{Area}$$ Equation (37)

For a perfectly fragmenting system with no apparent axial pressure $(2\pi r^2 \rightarrow 0)$, the radial pressure is assumed to be directly proportional to the strength of the compact, σ_c, and the maximum fragmenting applied force, F, is comparable to the crushing strength, C. Hence, combining Equations (36) and (37), we obtain:

$$\sigma = \frac{C}{\frac{\pi DT}{2}}$$ Equation (38)

For a compact with thickness, T, Equation (38) is then simplified into the relation:

$$\sigma_c = \frac{2C}{\pi DT} \qquad \text{Equation (39)}$$

From equation (39), σ_c was measured in kg/cm², crushing strength, C, was measured in kg, thickness and diameter were converted from inches to centimeters. Lubricity index is calculated from ratio of the difference between compact strengths of un-lubricated and lubricated material and the unlubricated material as shown by the relation:

$$\Omega = \frac{\sigma_{c,un\,lub\,ed} - \sigma_{c,lub\,ed}}{\sigma_{c,un\,lub\,ed}} x100 \qquad \text{Equation (40)}$$

Figure 14 shows the plots of average lubricity indices for the blends lubricated with various ratios of MgSt polymorphs (n=6; RSD <2.1%). Results from the lubricity evaluation show that MgSt-D (DD01) had the least tendency to cause over-lubrication (LI value: 5) compared to MsSt-M (DM01) with LI value of 6.25) and MgSt-A (DA01) with LI value of 12.5. The ranking for lowest tendency to cause blend over-lubrication at fixed concentration and lubrication time is as follows: DD01 < DM01 < D7 = D6 = D2 < DA01 < others. This ranking suggests that the level of water of hydration (or lack thereof) in the MgSt influences the tendency for over-lubrication.

This review found that the determination of lubricity index could be a great tool for the pre-formulation scientist. Is was observed that when LI values are over 10, reducing the amount of lubricant or lubrication time should be considered as effect of the lubricant on content uniformity and hardness might be exaggerated.

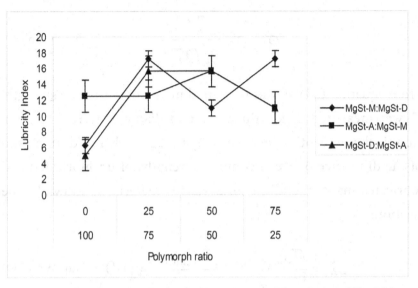

Figure 14: Average lubricity indices of various ratios MgSt Polymorphs (n=3; RSD <2.1%); MgSt-M:MgSt-D ratio means 100%:0% from left to right on x-axis; MgSt-A: MgSt-M ratio means 100%:0% from left to right on x-axis; and MgSt-D: MgSt-A ratio means 100%:0% from left to right on x-axis (Ref: PC Okoye, doctorate thesis).

3.2.8 Influence of Lubrication on Powder Mixtures

It is not usually possible to visualize the physical effect of lubrication during manufacturing process. One may observe densification on bench-top scale if very observant or when using plexi-glass blending apparatus. In order to review this influence of lubrication, we will use a few cases below.

Case 1: This case illustrates the changes that take place when lubrication of powder mixtures is monitored or visualized. The process was monitored using effusivity sensors (Mathis Instruments, Canada). Effusivity plots showed changes in powder density as (a) concentration of MgSt increases and (b) increasing mixing/lubrication time (Figure 15).

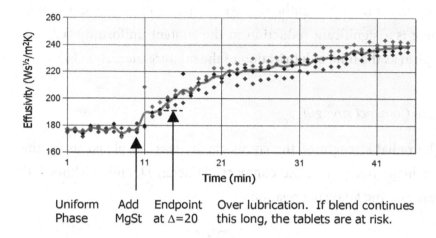

Uniform   Add   Endpoint   Over lubrication. If blend continues
Phase   MgSt   at Δ=20   this long, the tablets are at risk.

Figure 15: Effusivity sensors showing influence of lubrication (Reference: Mathis, Canada)

Another good way to visualize the influence of MgSt lubrication on powder mixtures is to measure the height or volume of the powder mixture on the blender pre-lubrication and post-lubrication (Figure 16). Notice that in the example below, the volume of powder mixture decreased at post-lubrication.

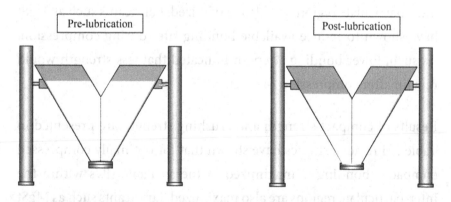

Figure 16: Pre-lubrication and post-lubrication schematic of v-blender containing powder mixture, indicating level of densification as a function of lubrication (Reference: Mathis, Canada)

Case 2: A statistical model demonstrated the presence of interaction between concentration of MgSt (undifferentiated form) and lubrication time. The authors observed that at a given concentration there is a significant reduction in the content uniformity (CU) of aspirin as the time of lubrication of the mixture increases [14].

3.2.6 Compact strength, σ_c

The radial strength of the compacts, σ_c, was calculated using the crushing strength, C, the compact diameter, D, and thickness, T, based on the following relation:

$$\sigma_c = \frac{2C}{\pi DT}$$

Equation (41)

From equation (41), σ_c was measured in kg/cm², crushing strength, C, was measured in kg, thickness and diameter were converted from inches to centimeters. All crushing strength values were obtained in triplicate. Previous studies have shown that for optimally compressed compacts, bonding was maximized as the available sites within the inter-particulate regions are also maximized. Lubricants such as MgSt have shown to reduce available bonding sites during compression. As such, lower bonding strength indicated that less strength would remain after compression [41-44].

Results of compact strength and crushing strength are presented in Table 7. Previous studies have shown that for optimally compressed compacts, bonding is maximized as the available sites within the inter-particulate regions are also maximized. Lubricants such as MgSt have shown to reduce available bonding sites during compression. As such, lower bonding strength would indicate that less strength would remain after compression [25, 28]. The results from compact strength show that the un-lubricated blend had the highest value of 15.471 kg/cm^2 followed by DD01 containing only MgSt-D with 14.585 kg/cm^2. Results also show that increase in compact strengths result to comparable increase in crushing strengths for the compacts. The average crushing strength for un-lubricated blends is 16.000 kg followed by the average crushing strength of 15.250 kg for DD01 compacts. The ranking is represented by: un-lubricated Compacts > DD01>DM01>D50/M50 > others.

Polymorph ratio	Formula	True density[1], ρ_{True}, g/ml	Bulk density[2], ρ_{Bulk}, g/ml	Tapped density[3], ρTap, g/ml	Stability Index[4] (SI)	Lubricity Index[a]	Compact strength, σ_c, (kg/cm²)[b]
A50/M50	D1	1.59	0.39	0.63	0.96	15.63	13.10
A25/M75	D2	1.60	0.39	0.64	0.99	11.00	13.68
A75/M25	D3	1.60	0.38	0.63	0.97	12.50	13.54
D50/A50	D4	1.59	0.37	0.62	0.94	15.63	13.30
D75/A25	D5	1.60	0.37	0.62	0.96	15.63	12.96
D25/A75	D6	1.58	0.37	0.63	0.94	11.00	13.88
D50/M50	D7	1.60	0.39	0.64	0.98	11.00	14.18
D75/M25	D8	1.60	0.39	0.64	0.96	17.19	12.58
D25/M75	D9	1.60	0.39	0.64	0.97	17.19	12.81
A100	DA01	1.60	0.39	0.64	0.93	12.50	13.64
M100	DM01	1.59	0.39	0.63	0.97	6.25	14.45
D100	DD01	1.60	0.38	0.62	0.93	5.00	14.59
Un-lubricated	n/a	n/a	0.37	0.71	0.83	n/a	15.47

[1] True density (n=5; RSD <0.01%); [2] Bulk density (n=3; RSD <3.4%); [3] Tapped density (n=4; RSD <2.5%; RSD for un-lubricated = 11.48%); [4] SI is a measure of powder flowability with a value of 1.00 as optimal

[a] Lubricity Index is a dimensionless number; [b] Compact strength as calculated from crushing strengths and compact dimension; n/a = not applicable

Table 7: Blends and Compacts Data (Ref: PC Okoye, doctorate thesis)

Chapter IV

*In this chapter, the reader is presented
with findings from compressional forces,
magnesium ion distribution, and
content uniformity*

4.0 Tablet Level Characterization: Compressional Forces

Compressed tablets containing MgSt polymorphs were produced from the powder mixtures and evaluated for hardness, compressional forces, ejection force, and distribution of magnesium particle on the tablet surface.

Tablet compression was performed using a 10-station instrumented press with data-acquisition capability (Natoli Engineering, St. Charles, Missouri). Target tablet weight of 500 mg and hardness of 8 kp was maintained. The only variable monitored in the process was the polymorphic forms of MgSt used as lubricants together with their physical mixtures. The pre-compression, main compression and ejection forces were monitored or measured to evaluate the level of such influence on tablet performance. The influence of lubricants such as MgSt on these compression indices with respect to tableting tooling, have been shown to have benefit in process control and formulation development [39-43].

4.1 Pre-compression, Main Compression, Ejection, and Total Forces

Results of the compression analysis in Figure 17 (Plots A-D) present the pre-compression, main compression, ejection and total compression forces as evaluated for tablets produced from various singular and mixed polymorphs. The total forces are the combination of pre-compression, main compression and ejection forces.

The results indicate that all 3 combinational ratios of MgSt-M and MgSt-D gave tableting forces with less variability. In fact, the MgSt-M and MgSt-D ratios compared well to the results from

single MgSt-M alone suggesting that the monolithic MgSt-M could have dominant influence on achieving stable compressional forces. Results from Plot A (pre-compression forces), Plot C (ejection forces), and Plot D (total compression forces) suggest that tablets with MgSt-A or MgSt-D alone tend to require less total forces during tableting (Figure 17). The results from the tableting forces also show that MgSt-D combinations with MgSt-A tend to require less total forces than MgSt-D combinations with MgSt-M. These observations suggest that the presence of MgSt-M in any combination require more ejection force, and also, tends to have adverse influence on the tableting performance.

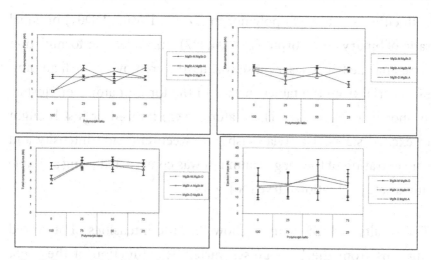

Figure 17: Compression Analysis - MgSt-M:MgSt-D ratio means 100%:0% from left to right on x-axis;
MgSt-A: MgSt-M ratio means 100%:0% from left to right on x-axis; and MgSt-D: MgSt-A ratio means 100%:0% from left to right on x-axis. Plot A shows the Pre-compression forces (n=10; RSD <11%); Plot B is the Main compression force (n=10; RSD <20%); Plot C is the Ejection force (n=10; RSD <48%); and Plot D shows the Total compression force (n=10; RSD <14%), Ref: PC Okoye, doctorate thesis.

4.2 Magnesium Ion Distribution on Tablet Surface

Previous study suggested that water permeation through capillaries in tablets depended on the concentration of MgSt, where higher proportions of the lubricant could cause an increase in the non-wetting internal surface resulting to an increasing number of capillaries not participating in water transport through the tablet [23]. In this study, Laser-induced breakdown spectroscopic analysis (LIBS) was performed on compressed tablets using PharmaLIBS™250 Version 1.32 (Pharmalaser, Quebec, Canada). LIBS technology is based on atomic emission spectroscopy (AES) of laser-produced plasma. Being a boundary lubricant, MgSt distribution on tablet surface layers was monitored based on Mg ion signal at wavelength of 518 nm. The laser was operated at 150 mJ with a repetition rate of 2 Hz and grating of 1200g/mm. Each camera has a delay of 0.8 μs and exposition of 5.0 μs. Six formulations selected for the LIBS analysis were lubricated with either single MgSt polymorph (DA01, DM01, DD01) or equal ratio of binary polymorphs (D1, D4, D7). Six tablets per formulation were analyzed. The laser pulse was used to remove a small amount of material from the tablet surface in the form of atoms or clusters as shown in Figure 17. These atoms were ionized or just brought to excited states. The relationship between emission intensity and concentration of the magnesium ion was constructed using a simple univariate calibration curve [46].

The results of LIBS analysis show that the intensities of atomized Mg ions from the laser pulses varied as a function of the MgSt polymorphs employed in the formulation. The intensity for DA01 was 35061 with RSD of 4.2%; the intensity of DM01 was 39260 with RSD of 3.1%; and the intensity of DD01 was 32187 with RSD of 3.3%. The intensities of 3 mixed ratios with equal contributions from each polymorph were also evaluated. The results show that D1 (A50:M50) has intensity of 37099 with RSD of 2.1%; the intensity of D4 (A50:D50) was found to be 31229 with RSD of 2.6%; and finally the intensity for D7 (M50:D50) was 35249 with RSD of 2.8%. These results show that blends lubricated with MgSt-M show the highest intensity, while blends lubricated with D50:A50 or MgSt-D have the lowest intensities (Figures 18A-D). The greatest signal intensity due to MgSt-M is believed to be related to its lower particle size distribution (d_{50} = 10.6 μm). The results also show minimal inter-tablet variability within the same formulation (n = 6; RSD < 5%). Analysis of variance performed using *Test for Equal Variances* showed the difference in particle distribution to be significant (p<0.005). The ranking for polymorphs with highest to lowest on laser intensity for Mg ion is: MgSt-M > D1 > D7 > MgSt-A > MgSt-D > D4.

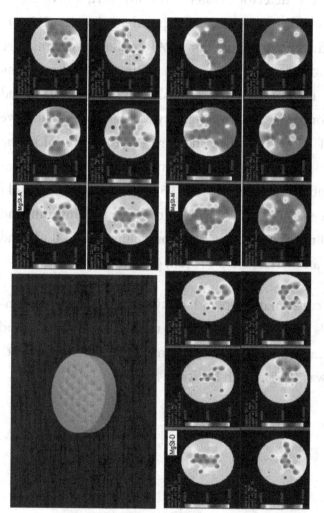

Clockwise: Figure 18 (A) Craters formed by the laser ablation at 37 sites on a tablet; 14 (B) Laser Image Mg-ion intensity for APAP tablets lubricated MgSt-A. The images show the levels of intensity of MgSt ion on the tablet surface; 14 (C) Laser Image of Mg-ion intensity for APAP tablets lubricated MgSt-M. The images indicate disproportionate (more clustering) distribution of Mg ion on the tablets lubricated with the monohydrate polymorph; 14 (D) Laser Image of Mg-ion intensity for APAP tablets lubricated MgSt-D showing lower clustering in terms of distribution of Mg ion on the tablets lubricated with the dihydrate polymorph (Ref: PC Okoye, doctorate thesis).

4.3 Content Uniformity

Drug substance assay in the powder mixture was analyzed using a high-performance liquid chromatographic unit (HPLC), Alliance 2695 with 2487 UV detector (Waters, Milford, MA, USA). Assay was performed on three pre-lubricated powder mixtures (D2, D3 and D4) to confirm homogeneity for APAP in the powder mixture or blend prior to lubrication. Powder samples (1 – 3 times) the unit-dose (500 - 1500 mg), were tested using an internally validated HPLC method for APAP. System suitability was conducted using five (5) injections of APAP reference standard (0.11018 mg/mL). The correlation coefficient (r^2) for each reference standard injection was >0.9999. The mobile phase consisted of 95 % Water / 5 % Methanol / 0.1% Trifluoroacetic Acid (TFA), with a flow rate of 1.0 mL/min and detection at 280 nm. The sample injection volume was 1.0 µL. and the column was an Inertsil, ODS-3, 5µm, 4.6 x 150mm.

Results of the confirmatory blend assay performed on the un-lubricated blends using a qualified HPLC method for APAP showed that the unlubricated powder mixture from batch D2 had an assay of 90%; batch D3 was 106%, batch D4 was 94%.

Chapter V

In this chapter, the reader is presented
with findings from dissolution studies,
solubility, tablet hardness, powder/particle
analysis, and suggested ingredient specifications

5.0 MgSt Polymorphs and Biopharmaceutic Classes II and III

Evaluation and review of the effect of MgSt polymorphs on the drug substances within the biopharmaceutics classes II and III were conducted using solubility and drug dissolution. Tablet hardness was also evaluated relative to the varying concentrations of the lubricants.

5.1 Prototype Formulation 2: Dissolution

Twelve-20 g formulations (including a control for each API without lubrication) were prepared in a mixer as shown on Table 8. Each formulation was blended for 4 minutes and then lubricated for 2 minutes. The composition of the control blend was: 20% API and 80% MCC. Direct compression blends employed in this experimentation contained:

5.1.1 APAP (20%); MCC (70 - 79%); and MgSt polymorphs (1%, 3%, 5%, 7%, 10%). Experimental design will show the various ratios of MgSt polymorphs to be used in the formulations. The amount of MCC diluent depended on the percent of MgSt polymorph used. All materials will be de-lumped prior to mixing.

5.1.2 NAPR (20%); MCC (70 - 79%); and MgSt polymorphs (1%, 3%, 5%, 7%, 10%). Experimental design will show the various ratios of MgSt polymorphs to be used in the formulations. The amount of MCC diluent depended on the percent of MgSt polymorph used. All materials will be de-lumped prior to mixing.

NAPR	MCC	MgSt[1]		APAP	MCC	MgSt[2]
% w/w				% w/w		
20	79	1		20	79	1
20	77	3		20	77	3
20	75	5		20	75	5
20	73	7		20	73	7
20	70	10		20	70	10
[1]Percent of MgSt polymorph in the powder mixture (BCS II);						
[2]Percent of MgSt polymorph in the powder mixture (BCS III)						

Table 8: Experimental Designs - MgSt Polymorphs and BCS II & III (Ref: PC Okoye, doctorate thesis)

The *in vitro* dissolution for immediate-release (IR) solid-dosage forms often follows first-order process for solid as proposed by Noyes-Whitney in the relation:

$$\frac{dW}{dt} = kS(C_s - C_t)$$ Equation (42)

Where $\frac{dW}{dt}$ is the amount of drug dissolved per unit time; C_t is the drug concentration (mg/mL) at a given time; C_s is the saturated solubility or concentration (mg/mL); k is the dissolution rate constant (cm.min^{-1}); S represents the surface area of the solid; and t is the time (sec). k is also represented by D/h where D is diffusion coefficient (cm^2.min^{-1}); and h is the thickness (cm) of the diffusion layer [28, 39].

In this study, *in vitro* dissolution for immediate-release (IR) solid-dosage forms of APAP and NAPR was conducted using USP 30 Apparatus 2 (Paddle Apparatus) in 900 ml of phosphate buffer solution at 37 ±0.5 ºC and at a rotational speed of 50 rpm [42]. Dissolution samples were withdrawn at predetermined intervals and filtered through 0.45 mm filters. The drug assay for APAP was determined spectrophotometrically directly at λmax of 243 nm, using phosphate butter at pH 5.8. Standard calibration curve for APAP was developed using phosphate buffer solution at pH of 5.8 and λmax of 243 nm. Drug assay for NAPR was determined spectrophotometrically directly at λmax of 271 nm, using phosphate butter at pH 7.4. Standard calibration curve for NAPR was developed using phosphate buffer solution at pH of 7.4 and λmax of 271 nm. All UV-VIS spectrophotometric analysis was conducted using UV-VIS Spectrophotometer PharmaSpec UV-1700 (Shimadzu, Japan) and a Dissolution apparatus, USP 30 Paddle Apparatus #2 (Distek, North Brunswick, NJ) [48].

5.2 Solubility

Solubility studies were conducted using excess amounts of the active ingredients. Spectrophotometric analysis follows Beer's Law of absorption as given by:

$$A = \log \frac{1}{T} = abc \qquad \text{Equation (43)}$$

Where A is Absorbance; T is transmittance; a is absorptivity; b is pathlength (cm); and c is concentration (M) [47].

5.2.1 Acetaminophen (APAP)

Aqueous solubility of 14.3 mg/mL at 25 °C. A log P (n-octanol/water) value of 0.2 has been measured. An acidic pKa of 9.5 at 25 °C is reported [29]. For this study, a super-saturated solution of APAP will be prepared using five grams (5g) of APAP in 100 ml of De-ionized Water. The suspension will be sonicated for 60 minutes and sampled at intervals of 0, 4, 8, 24 hours, and 72 hours for equilibrium solubility studies. The supernatant will be filtered at isothermal conditions. The equilibrium concentrations will be determined by measuring absorbance after appropriate dilutions and interpolations. The samples will be analyzed using UV-VIS Spectrophotometer PharmaSpec UV-1700 (Shimadzu, Japan). Standard calibration curve will be developed using phosphate buffer solution at pH of 5.8 and λmax of 243 [48].

5.2.2 Naproxen (NAPR)

Aqueous solubility of 15.9 mcg/mL at 25 °C. A log P (n-octanol/water) value of 2.8 has been measured. An acidic pKa of 4.2 at 25 °C is reported [28, 49]. For this study, a super-saturated suspension of NAPR will be prepared using twenty milligrams (20 mg) of NAPR in 50 mL of De-ionized Water. The suspension will be sonicated for 60 minutes and sampled at intervals of 0, 4, 8, 24 hours, and 72 hours for equilibrium solubility studies. The supernatant will be filtered at isothermal conditions. The equilibrium concentrations will be determined by measuring absorbance after appropriate dilutions and interpolations. All the samples will be analyzed using UV-VIS Spectrophotometer PharmaSpec UV-1700 (Shimadzu, Japan). Standard calibration curve will be developed using phosphate buffer solution at pH of 7.4 and λmax of 271 [48].

5.3 Hardness of APAP Tablets Lubricated with MgSt Polymorphs

Results of the hardness analysis for APAP tablets lubricated with are shown in Figure 19. The results showed comparable hardness values for APAP tablets when lubricant concentration was the same for the polymorphs. As expected, the un-lubricated (control) tablets (%RSD = 0.82) showed higher hardness than lubricated tablets. Generally, tablets lubricated with 5% or more MgSt showed lower hardness below 20 kp and could affect tablet dissolution significantly [53, 54, 55]. Tablet hardness was found to decrease with increasing lubricant concentration. Analysis using *Paired T-Test* showed that this difference between lubricated and un-lubricated tablets was significant (p<0.005). Similarly, statistically significant differences were observed in hardness values between MgSt-A and MgSt-D (p<0.005); and MgSt-A and MgSt-M (p<0.005), but not between MgSt-M vs MgSt-D (p>0.224).

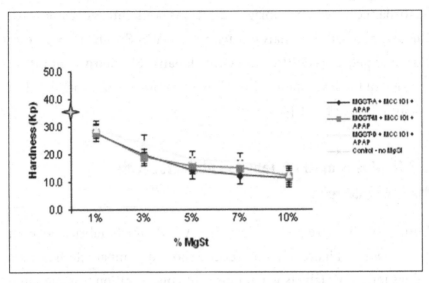

Figure 19: Hardness of APAP tablets lubricated MgSt Polymorphs. The plots showed the differences in tablet hardness as a function of lubricant concentration (Ref: PC Okoye, doctorate thesis).

5.4 Hardness of NAPR Tablets Lubricated with MgSt Polymorphs

Results of the hardness analysis for NAPR tablets lubricated with are depicted in Figure 20. The results showed comparable hardness values for NAPR tablets when lubricant concentration was the same for the polymorphs. The control (un-lubricated) tablets (%RSD = 0.3) also showed higher hardness than lubricated tablets. Analysis using *Paired T-Test* showed that this difference between lubricated and un-lubricated tablets was significant (p<0.007). Tablet hardness was found to decrease with increasing lubricant concentration. Similarly, statistically significant differences were observed in hardness values between MgSt-A and MgSt-D (p<0.005); and MgSt-A and MgSt-M (p<0.005), but not between MgSt-M vs MgSt-D (p>0.325).

It is worth-noting that the hardness values for NAPR tablets were less impacted by lubrication than the APAP tablets. This could mean that a model BCS Class II may exhibit higher hardness than BCS model Class III drug. This finding was demonstrated by the results from the data analysis using *Paired T-Test*, which showed statistical difference between the hardness values between lubricated and un-lubricated tablets (APAP with p<0.005; NAPR with p<0.012).

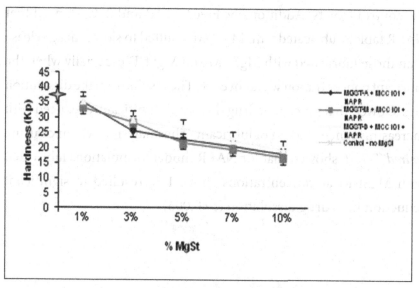

Figure 20: Hardness of NAPR tablets lubricated MgSt Polymorphs. The plots showed the differences in tablet hardness as a function of lubricant concentration (Ref: PC Okoye, doctorate thesis).

Tablet hardness for MgSt polymorphs illustrated the unique similarities in their performance during tablet compression. The polymorphs performed comparably in terms of effects on tablet hardness within the same concentration. However, it also demonstrated the deleterious effect of high concentration of lubricants on tablet hardness. Analysis using *Paired T-Test* showed that lubricant concentration above 3% had significant impact on tablet hardness by interfering with tablet tensile strength (p<0.005). The hardness of tablets decreased with increasing lubricant concentration.

5.5 Dissolution of NAPR Tablets Lubricated with MgSt Polymorphs

Results from NAPR tablet dissolution are presented in Figures 21 (A, B, C). The result pointed to difference in behavior of the MgSt polymorphs with respect to the BCS II (NAPR) model drug. The Figure 21A showed that the dissolution of NAPR tablets lubricated with 1% to 3% MgSt-A compared well to the dissolution profile of the control tablets. Additionally, Figures 21B and 21C, showed that NAPR tablets lubricated with MgSt-M resulted to slower drug release than those lubricated with MgSt-M and MgSt-D especially when the lubricant concentration was above 1%. The results from the dissolution also showed that percent of drug dissolved significantly reduced with increasing concentration of lubricant. The analysis of variance using *Paired T-Test*, showed that for NAPR model formulations lubricated with MgSt-M at concentrations above 1 % resulted to significant reduction in % drug dissolution ($p < 0.005$).

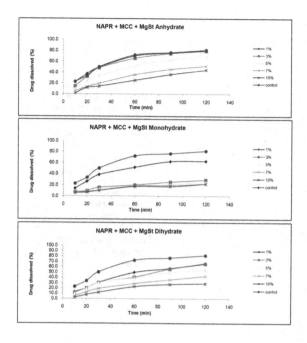

Figure 21 (A): Dissolution Profile of NAPR tablets lubricated MgSt Anhydrate. The plots showed the differences in tablet dissolution as a function of lubricant concentration.; Figure 20 B: Dissolution Profile of NAPR tablets lubricated MgSt Monohydrate. The plots showed the differences in tablet dissolution as a function of lubricant concentration.; Figure 20 C: Dissolution Profile of NAPR tablets lubricated MgSt Dihydrate. The plots showed the differences in tablet dissolution as a function of lubricant concentration. (Ref: PC Okoye, doctorate thesis).

5.6 Dissolution of APAP Tablets Lubricated with MgSt Polymorphs

The results from the dissolution study using APAP tablets are presented in Figures 22 (A, B, C). The result showed that APAP tablets lubricated with 1% to 10% MgSt-D resulted to much slower drug release than those lubricated with equal concentrations of MgSt-M (MgSt-D vs MgSt-M: $p<0.005$); and MgSt-A (MgSt-D vs MgSt-A: $p<0.005$). This result seemed to suggest that when used at equal concentrations, MgSt-D polymorph had much greater retarding effect on dissolution of immediate release tablets in BCS Class III when compared to MgSt-A and MgSt-M. Hence, in order to elicit the same dissolution profile or response, a much lower concentration (<1%) may be appropriate for MgSt-D.

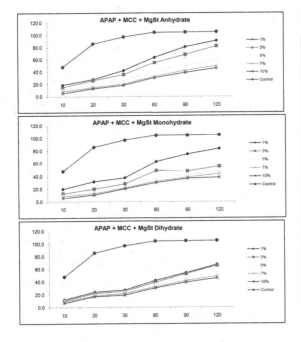

Figure 22 (A, B, C) Dissolution Profile of APAP tablets lubricated MgSt Anhydrate. The plots showed the differences in tablet dissolution as a function of lubricant concentration. Figure 21B: Dissolution Profile of APAP tablets lubricated MgSt Monohydrate. The plots showed the differences in tablet dissolution as a function of lubricant concentration. Figure 21C: Dissolution Profile of APAP tablets lubricated MgSt Dihydrate. The plots showed the differences in tablet dissolution as a function of lubricant concentration. (Ref: PC Okoye, doctorate thesis)

5.7 Retarding Effect of MgSt Polymorphs on Dissolution of Model Drugs

Figures 23 and 24 showed the comparative analysis of retarding effect on dissolution based on the type and level of lubricant in the formulation. The plot for BCS Class II Model drug, NAPR, showed that at 1% level, MgSt-M produced the same retarding effect on dissolution as 3% MgSt-D and 5% MgSt-A. On the other hand, and for BCS Class III model drug, APAP, at 1% level, MgSt-D produced the same retarding effect on dissolution as 3% MgSt-M and 5% MgSt-A.

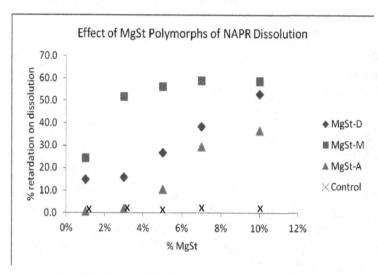

Figure 23: Retarding Effect of % MgSt Polymorphs on BCS Class II Model Drug. The plot depicted the extent of dissolution retardation based on type of lubricant as compared to the Control (non-lubricated), Ref: PC Okoye, doctorate thesis.

For BCS II model drug, NAPR, with high permeability and low solubility characteristics, MgSt-A had much similar profile as the control tablet. However, the negative effect was much less compared to higher deleterious effect on drug dissolution by MgSt-M. Figure 23 showed the comparative analysis of type of lubricant and level of lubrication on dissolution profile of immediate release tablets. MgSt-M produced the most retarding effect on dissolution as compared to MgSt-A and MgSt-D. The analysis of variance (ANOVA) showed that the significance of this finding is that the potential to over-lubricating the model drug, NAPR, is higher when MgSt-M is employed as lubricant ($p<0.005$). This can be explained by the high interfacial tension between the MgSt-M – moisture (217.2 dyne cm^{-1}) and the low solubility of the model drug, NAPR.

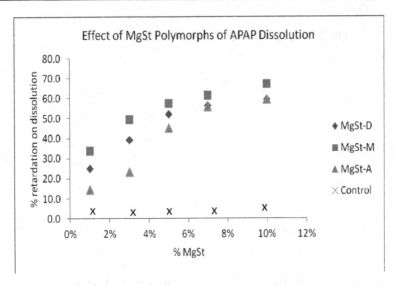

Figure 24: Retarding Effect of % MgSt Polymorphs on BCS Class III Model Drug. The plot depicted the extent of dissolution retardation based on type of lubricant as compared to the Control (non-lubricated), Ref: PC Okoye, doctorate thesis.

With regards to BCS Class III model drug, APAP with high solubility and low permeability, Figure 24 showed that MgSt-M produced the most retarding effect on dissolution as compared to MgSt-A and MgSt-D. Here, the potential to over-lubricating the model drug, APAP, is highest when MgSt-M is employed as lubricant. This can be explained by the high interfacial tension between the MgSt-M – moisture (217.2 dyne cm^{-1}) and the low permeability of the model drug, APAP.

Overall, for BCS Class II (NAPR) & Class III (APAP) model drugs, tablets lubricated with MgSt monohydrate showed highest % retardation to dissolution (than MgSt-A & MgSt-D) when compared to non-lubricated tablets. This effect could be related to higher interfacial tension for the MgSt-M compared to MgSt-A and MgSt-D. Additionally, the water of hydration appeared to be tightly bound in the MgSt-M (as observed from DSC trace) compared to MgSt-D and may not be readily available for dissolution.

5.8 Effect of MgSt Polymorphs on Dissolution Rate Constant, k

In vitro drug dissolution for immediate release tablets follows first-order kinetics based on the assumption of sink condition and saturated solubility concentration for the drug substance. Table 9 shows the results for estimated mean dissolution rate constant, *k*, as derived from the dissolution rate using the Noyes-Whitney Equation (Equation 42). The effect of lubricant concentration on dissolution rate was estimated using 1-5% concentration of the MgSt polymorphs. The rates of *in vitro* drug dissolution for the BCS Class II and III model drugs were calculated based on the lubricant concentration, the amount of drug dissolved from the tablets, the mean surface area of tablet (5.985 cm^2), and saturated drug solubility at 25 °C.

The mean dissolution rate constant for naproxen lubricated with MgSt-A was found to be 7.0 x10^{-3} cm.min^{-1} compared to 4.0 x10^{-3} cm.min^{-1} for MgSt-M and 6.0 x10^{-3} cm.min^{-1} for MgSt-D. The mean dissolution rate constant for acetaminophen lubricated with MgSt-A was found to be 6.6 x10^{-3} cm.min^{-1} compared to 5.0 x10^{-3} cm.min^{-1} for MgSt-M and 5.5x10^{-3} cm.min^{-1} for MgSt-D.

The results showed that MgSt anhydrate had the least negative impact on rate of *in vitro* drug dissolution for both BCS Classes II and III compared to MgSt-M and MgSt-D. This behavior can be explained by the absence of water of hydration which makes the anhydrate form more susceptible to the *random walk* phenomenon wherein the pores acts in capillary manner to imbibe dissolution media and create an increase in wettability.

The results from dissolution rate constant also showed that the BCS Class II model drug (NAPR) had higher rate constant than the BCS Class III model drug (APAP). This phenomenon can be explained by the greater lipophilicity (higher permeability) of the BCS Class II drugs, which provides a lower barrier for lubricants like MgSt that possesses long chain fatty acids than for BCS Class III drugs with lower lipophilicity.

BCS Class II Drug Dissolution (Naproxen Tablets IR)			
	Lubricant concentration (1 – 5%)		
	MgSt-A	MgSt-M	MgSt-D
Mean Dissolution Rate Constant, k (cm.min^{-1})	7.0×10^{-3}	4.0×10^{-3}	6.0×10^{-3}
Standard Deviation	0.001	0.002	0.001
BCS Class III Drug Dissolution (Acetaminophen Tablets IR)			
	Lubricant concentration (1 - 5%)		
	MgSt-A	MgSt-M	MgSt-D
Mean Dissolution Rate Constant, k (cm.min^{-1})	6.6×10^{-3}	5.0×10^{-3}	5.5×10^{-3}
Standard Deviation	0.001	0.002	0.001

Table 9: Effect of MgSt Polymorphs on Dissolution Rate (Ref: PC Okoye, doctorate thesis)

Appendix 1: Overall Ranking for MgSt Polymorph Ratios Based on Good, Fair, and Poor Performance

Formula	MgSt Ratio	LI	porosity	Permea-bility	% comp	Stability Index	δ-effusivity	Pre-comp force	Main comp force	Ejection force	LIBS	Good (G)	Fair (F)	Poor (P)	(5G + 3F) - P	Overall ranking*
D1	A50/M50	P	P	P	G	G	P	F	F	P	P	2	2	6	10	12th
D2	A25/M75	F	P	P	G	G	F	P	G	P		3	2	4	17	8th
D3	A75/M25	F	F	P	G	G	F	P	G	F		3	4	2	25	6th
D4	D50/A50	P	G	P	G	G	G	P	G	G	F	6	1	3	30	4th
D5	D75/A25	P	G	F	G	G	G	F	G	G		6	2	1	35	2nd
D6	D25/A75	F	G	F	G	G	P	F	P	G		4	3	2	27	5th
D7	D50/M50	F	F	P	G	G	P	F	P	P	P	2	3	5	14	10th
D8	D75/M25	P	P	P	G	G	G	F	F	F		3	3	3	21	7th
D9	D25/M75	P	P	P	G	G	P	F	F	F		2	3	4	15	9th
DA01	MgSt-A	F	F	G	F	G	P	G	F	G	F	4	5	1	34	3rd
DM01	MgSt-M	G	P	P	G	G	P	F	P	P	P	3	1	6	12	11th
DD01	MgSt-D	G	F	G	G	G	G	G	F	G	G	8	2	0	46	1st

* Overall ranking ≥ 20 appears to suggest acceptable performance

LI = Lubricity Index

LIBS = Laser-induced Breakdown Spectroscopy

Ref: PC Okoye, doctorate thesis

Appendix 2: Magnesium Stearate Specifications

Proposed Specifications: Magnesium Stearate Polymorphs

Product Code	MgSt (mixed form)*	MgSt Anhydrous	MgSt Monohydrate	MgSt Dihydrate
Stearic: Palmitic	65:35	65:35	65:35	65:35
Particle Size, 50th %	10.5-16.5 microns	10.0-15.5 microns	10.0-15.5 microns	10.0-15.5 microns
Particle Size, 90th %	35 micron max	35 micron max	35 micron max	35 micron max
Specific Surface Area	2 - 15 m^2/g**	5-10 m^2/g	5-10 m^2/g	5-10 m^2/g
Apparent Density	0.08-0.17 g/cc	0.08-0.17 g/cc	0.08-0.17 g/cc	0.08-0.17 g/cc
Interfacial tension,	Unknown	150-240 dyne cm^{-1}	50-90 dyne cm^{-1}	30-70 dyne cm^{-1}
Loss on drying	<<6.0%	2-6%	3-5%	4-6%
Bound water	Unknown	<0.5%	~2.88%	~5.56%
Water activity (25°C)	Unknown	0.25-0.45	0.25-0.45	0.25-0.45
Free Fatty Acid	2.0% max	2.0% max	2.0% max	2.0% max
Assay (MgO) (FCC)	6.8-8.3%	6.8-8.3%	6.8-8.3%	6.8-8.3%
Appearance	Fine, white powder	Fine, white powder	Fine, white powder	Fine, white powder
ID (Magnesium)	Meets requirement	Meets requirement	Meets requirement	Meets requirement

*Mixed form conforms to FCC requirements
** Typical specific surface area
References: (1) Mallinckrodt, Inc.; (2) Handbook of Pharmaceutical Excipients 4th edition. London: Pharmaceutical Press;
(3) Ref: PC Okoye, doctorate thesis

Appendix 3: Current Structure for MgSt

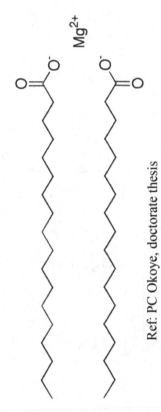

Ref: PC Okoye, doctorate thesis

Appendix 4: Proposed Structure for MgSt monohydrate

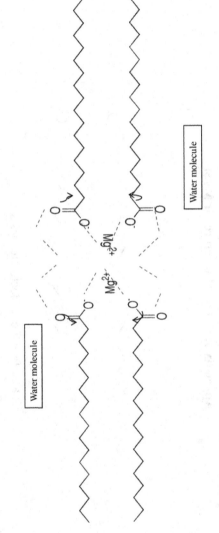

Water molecule

Water molecule

Ref: PC Okoye, doctorate thesis

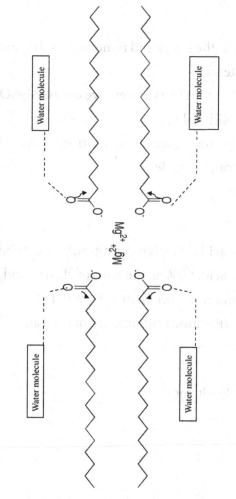

Appendix 5: Proposed Structure for MgSt dihydrate

Ref: PC Okoye, doctorate thesis

SYNTHESIS OF MAGNESIUM STEARATE

$C_{17}H_{35}COOH^* + NaOH \to C_{17}H_{35}COONa + H2O$

$2C_{17}H_{35}COONa + MgSO_4 7H2O \to Mg(C_{17}H_{35}COO)_2 \cdot H2O + Na_2SO_4 + 6H2O$

- Add water to the slurry and remove the soluble salts and drain off the water.
- Adjust pH of the slurry to remove excess $MgSO_4$.
- Separate solid and dry.
- Depending on reaction conditions, monohydrate and dihydrate can be made.

* Stearic acid

- Stearic acid (USP/NF definition) – Contains at least 40% stearic acid, 90% as the sum of stearic acid and palmitic acid, and not more than 6.0% water.
- Stearic/Palmitic acid mixture may be animal or vegetable origin.

(Reference: Mallinckrodt, Inc)

Glossary

MgSt	Magnesium stearate
MgSt-A	Magnesium stearate anhydrous
MgSt-M	Magnesium stearate monohydrate
MgSt-D	Magnesium stearate dihydrate
DA01	Neat Magnesium stearate anhydrous
DD01	Neat Magnesium stearate dihydrate
DM01	Neat Magnesium stearate monohydrate
TCi	Thermal Conductivity
FT-IR	Fourier Transform Infra Red Spectroscopy
pXRD	Powder X-Ray Diffraction
TGA	Thermogravimetry
BCS	Biopharmaceutic Classification System
DSC	Differential Scanning Calorimetry
DVS	Dynamic Vapor Sorption
LIBS	Laser-induced breakdown spectroscopy
APAP	Acetaminophen
NAPR	Naproxen
MCC	Microcrystalline cellulose
LAC-M	Lactose monohydrate
BFE	Basic flowability energy
SI	Stability Index

Ω	Lubricity Index (LI)
BET	Brunauer, Emmett, Teller
ΔE	Surface binding energy
γ	Interfacial tension
a_w	Water Activity
ϵ_{Total}	Total Porosity
ΔH_{vap}	Heat of Vaporization (Enthalpy)
ρ_{True}	True Density
ε_{Total}	Total Porosity
σ_c	Compact strength
m_0	Monolayer content
C	Binding Constant
K	Kelvin
°C	Celcius
ΔG	Change in Gibbs Energy
API	Active Pharmaceutical Ingredient
R	Gas Constant
%RSD	Percent Relative Standard Deviation
R^2	Linearity
USP	United States Pharmacopeia

Bibliography

1. Okoye P, Wu HS, Dave RH. (2012). To Evaluate the Effect of Various Magnesium Stearate Polymorphs using Powder Rheology and Thermal Analysis. Drug Development and Industrial Pharmacy. 38 (12), 1470 – 1478.
2. Stallings A (2005). Approach to Understanding Immediate Release Dosage Forms: Dissolution Failures due to Effects of Magnesium Stearate in Pharmaceutical Formulations. AAPS Poster W4332.
3. Arratia P, Muzzio F (2006). Characterizing Mixing and Lubrication in the Bohle Bin Blender. Powder Technol. 161, 202–208.
4. Turkoglu M, Sahin I, San T (2005). Evaluation of Hexagonal Boron Nitride as a New Tablet Lubricant. J. Pharm. Dev. Technol. 10 (3), 381–388.
5. Lieberman H, Lachman L, Schwartz J (1989). Pharmaceutical Dosage Forms: Tablets Vol. 1 (Marcel Dekker, New York, 2d ed.), pp. 195–246.
6. Nichols AG (2008). Magnesium Anhydrate Report, Corporate Analytical Research, Mallinckrodt Pharmaceutical, Inc.
7. Nichols AG, Wu HS. (2008). Characterization of Stearate-based Lubricants for Making Tablets. AAPS Poster No. T3218, AM-08-00825.

8. Okoye P, Wu HS. (2007). Lubrication of Direct-Compressible Blends with Magnesium Stearate Monohydrate and Dihydrate. Pharm. Technol. 13:116 – 129.

9. Patel S, Kaushal AM, Bansal AK. (2007). Lubrication Potential of Magnesium Stearate Studied on Instrumented Rotary Tablet Press. AAPS PharmSciTech 8 (4) Article 89: E1-8, http://www.aapspharmscitech.org.

10. International Cosmetic Ingredient Dictionary and Handbook. (2008). Cosmetic, Toiletry and Fragrance Association (CTFA) Twelfth Ed.

11. Young PM, Traini D. (2007). Advances in Pulmonary Therapy. Drug and the Pharm. Sci. 172:16.

12. Ertel KD, Cartensen JT. (1988). Chemical, Physical, and Lubricant Properties of Magnesium Stearate. J. Pharm. Sci. 77 (7): 625 – 629.

13. Sharpe SA, Celik M, Newman AW, Brittain HG. (1997). Physical Characterization of the Polymorphic Variations of Magnesium Stearate and Magnesium Palmitate Hydrate Species. Struct. Chem. 8:73-74.

14. Swaminathan V, Kildsig DO. (2002). Effect of Magnesium Stearate on the Content Uniformity of Active Ingredient in Pharmaceutical Powder Mixtures. AAPS PharmSciTech 3 (3) article 19:1-5.

15. Koivisto M, Jalonen HU, Lehto V. (2004). Effect of Temperature and Humidity on Vegetable Grade of Magnesium Stearate. Powder Technol. 147:79-85.

16. Leinonen UI, Jalonen HU, Vihervaara PA, Laine ESU. (1992). Physical and Lubrication Properties of Magnesium Stearate. J. Pharm. Sci. 81 (12):1194-1198.

17. Steffens KJ, Koglin J. (1993). The Magnesium Stearate Problem. Manuf. Chem. Dec. 1993:16-18.

18. Andres C, Bracconi P, Pourcelot Y. (2001). On the Difficulty of Assessing the Specific Surface Area of Magnesium Stearate. Int J Pharm 218:153-163.

19. Bracconi P, Andres C, Ndiaye A. (2003). Structural Properties of Magnesium Stearate Pseudopolymorphs: Effect of Temperature. Int J Pharm 262:109-124.

20. Swaminathan V, Kildsig DO. (2001). An Examination of the Moisture Sorption Characteristics of Commercial Magnesium Stearate. AAPS PharmSciTech 2 (4) article 28:1-7.

21. Almaya A, Aburub A. (2008). Effect of Particle Size on Compaction of Materials with Different Deformation Mechanisms with and without Lubricants. AAPS PharmSciTech 9 (2):414-418.

22. Shah RB, Tawakkaul MA, Khan MA. (2008). Comparative Evaluation of Flow for Pharmaceutical Powders and Granules. AAPS PharmSciTech 9 (1):250-258.

23. Ganderton D. (1969). The Effect of Distribution of Magnesium Stearate on the Permeation of a Tablet by Water. J Pharm Pharmac. 21 (Suppl):9S-18S.

24. Barra J, Somma R. (1996). Influence of the Physicochemical Variability of Magnesium Stearate on its Lubricant Properties: Possible Solutions. Drug Dev and Ind Pharm. 22 (11): 1105-1120.

25. Center for Drug Evaluation and Research (2000). Guidance for Industry - Waiver of In Vivo Bioavailability Studies for Immediate-Release Solid Oral Dosage Forms Based on a Biopharmaceutics Classification System. http://www.fda.gov/cder/guidance/index.htm, 1-13.

26. Yu LX, Amidon GL, Polli JE, Zhao H, Mehta MU, Conner DP, Shah VP, Lesko LJ, Chen M, Lee VHL, Hussain AS. (2002). Biopharmaceutic Classification System: The Scientific Basis for Biowaiver Extension. Pharm. Res. 19 (7): 921-925.

27. Bruttin F (2006). Where's the Business Case? Identifying and Articulating the Value Proposition for Institutionalizing PAT in Development and Manufacturing. Process Analytical Technology, Institute of Validation. www.ivthome.com.

28. Wilson W, Peng Y, Augsburger LL. (2005). Comparison of Statistical Analysis and Bayesian Networks in the Evaluation of Dissolution Performance of BCS Class II Model Drugs. J. Pharm. Sci. 94 (12): 2764-2776.

29. Kalantzi L, Reppas C, Dressman JB, Amidon GL, Junginger HE, Midha KK, Shah VP, Stavchansky SA, Barends DM. (2006). Biowaiver Monographs for Immediate Release Solid Oral Dosage Forms: Acetaminophen (Paracetamol). J. Pharm. Sci. 95 (1): 4-14.

30. Fundamentals of Moisture Sorption Isotherms. (2012). Application Notes, Decagon Devices. www.decagon.com.

31. Young PM, Edge S, Staniforth JN, Steele DF, Price R. (2005). Dynamic Vapor Sorption Properties of Sodium Starch Glycolate Disintegrants. Pharm. Dev. and Tech. (10) 249-259.

32. Kablan T, Clement YY, Francoise KA, Mathias OK. (2008). Determination and Modeling of Moisture Sorption Isotherms of Chitosan and Chitin. Act Chim. Slov. (55): 677-682.

33. Atkins, PW (1994). Physical Chemistry 5th edition. New York: W. H. Freeman and Company.

34. Freeman, R. (2007). Measuring the flow properties of consolidated, conditioned and aerated powders — A comparative study using a powder rheometer and a rotational shear cell. Powder Technol. 174 (1-2) 25-33.

35. Cooke J, Freeman R. (2006). The Flowability of Powders and Effect of Flow Additives. World Congress on Particle Tech. (5) 1-12.

36. Brittain HG. (1995). Physical Characterization of Pharmaceutical Solids. Marcel Dekker, Inc. 70 (9): 253-300.

37. Martin A, Bustamante P, Chun AHC. (1993). Physical Pharmacy: Physical Chemical Principles in the Pharmaceutical Sciences. Lea & Febiger, Fourth Ed.:423- 452.

38. Sun CC. (2008). Mechanism of Moisture Induced Variations in True Density and Compaction Properties of Microcrystalline Cellulose. Intl J. Pharm. 346: 93-101.

39. Lieberman H, Lachman L, Schwartz JB. (1990). Pharmaceutical Dosage Forms: Tablets. Marcel Dekker, Inc. (Vol. 2): 201-243.

40. Javadzadeh Y, Shariati H, Movahhed-Danesh E, Nokkodchi A. (2009). Effect of Some Commercial Grades of Microcrystalline Cellulose on Flowability, Compressibility, and Dissolution Profile of Piroxicam Liquisolid Compacts. Drug Dev and Ind Pharm. 35 (2): 243 - 251.

41. Busignies V, Leclerc B, Truchon S, Tchoreloff P. (2011). Changes in the Specific Surface Area of Tablets Composed of Pharmaceutical Materials with Various Deformation Behaviors. Drug Dev and Ind Pharm. 37 (2): 225 - 233.

42. Abdel-Hamid S, Betz G. (2011). Study of Radial Die-wall Pressure Changes during Pharmaceutical Powder Compaction. Drug Dev and Ind Pharm. 37 (4): 387 - 395.

43. Muzikova J, Eimerava I. (2011). A Study of the Compaction Process and the Properties of Tablets Made of a New Co-processed Starch Excipient. Drug Dev and Ind Pharm. 37 (5): 576 – 582.

44. Perrault M, Bertrand F, Chaouki J. (2001). An Experimental Investigation of the Effect of the Amount of Lubricant on Tablet Properties. Drug Dev and Ind Pharm. 37 (2): 234 – 242.

45. Weber D, Pu Y, Cooney C. (2008). Quantification of Lubricant Activity of Magnesium Stearate by Atomic Force Microscopy. Drug Dev and Ind Pharm. 34 (10): 1097 – 1099.

46. Sigman ME, Meintee EM, Bridge C. 2006. Application of Laser-Induced Breakdown Spectroscopy to Forensic Science: Analysis of Paint Samples. Award Number 2006-DN-BX-K251, Document Number 237839, National Center for Forensic Science and Dept of Chemistry, University of Central Florida, pp 1-84.

47. Connors KA. 1982. A Textbook of Pharmaceutical Analysis. Wiley-Interscience. 3rd Ed., 173 – 234.

48. USP Monographs, USP 35 NF 30. (2012). United States Pharmacopeia, National Formulary (1-3).

49. Mora CP, Martinez F. (2007). Solubility of Naproxen in Several Organic Solvents at Different Temperatures. Fluid Phase Equilibria. 255 (1): 70-77.

50. Rowe RC, Sheskey PJ, Weller PJ (2003). Handbook of Pharmaceutical Excipients 4th edition. London: Pharmaceutical Press.

51. Thomas MA. (2005). Magnesium Stearate: Solving the Surface Area Problem. *www.quantachrome.com/articles_pdf/magnesium.*

52. Sing KSW, Everett DH, Haul RA, Moscou L, Pierotti RA, Rouquerol J, Siemeniewska T. (1985). Reporting Physisorption Data for Gas/Solid Systems with Reference to the Determination of Surface Area and Porosity. Pure and Appl Chem., Vol 57 (4) 603 – 619.

53. Johnson JR, Wang L, Gordon MS, Chowhan ZT. (1991). Effect of Formulation Solubility and Hygroscopicity on Disintegrant Efficiency in Tablets Prepared by Wet Granulation in Terms of Dissolution. J. Pharm. Sci., 80 (5): 469-471.

54. Iranloye TA, Parrott EL. (1978). Effects of Compression force, Particle Size, and Lubricants on Dissolution Rate. J. Pharm. Sci., 67 (4): 535-539.

55. Levy G, Gumtow RH. (1963). Effect of Certain Tablet Formulation Factors on Dissolution Rate of the Active Ingredient III. Tablet Lubricants. J. Pharm. Sci., 52:1139-1144. Doi:10.1002/jps.2600521209.

56. Brunauer S, Emmett PH, Teller E. 1938. Adsorption of Gases in Multimolecular Layers. J. Am. Chem. Soc. 60 (2), 309-319.

Index

Printed in the United States
By Bookmasters

Printed in the United States
By Bookmasters